Fibromyalgia

Fibromyalgia

Simple Relief
through Movement

Stacie L. Bigelow, M.A.

John Wiley & Sons, Inc.
New York • Chichester • Weinheim • Brisbane • Singapore • Toronto

Published by John Wiley & Sons, Inc.
Published simultaneously in Canada

This publication is designed to provide accurate and authoritative information in
regard to the subject matter covered. It is sold with the understanding that the
publisher is not engaged in rendering professional services. If professional advice
or other expert assistance is required, the services of a competent professional
person should be sought.

ISBN 0-471-34802-3

To my parents.

For their ongoing gifts of life, love, and loyalty.

Contents

Preface

It's 9:30 A.M. on a cool, late September Saturday morning. Before I open my eyes, I try to stretch my heavy arms and legs. My muscles communicate their familiar protest to being stretched and resist my efforts. I let out a morning moan, which gets the attention of my housemate, who is already up and making breakfast. She peeks into the room and asks me how I feel. We have been through this conversation so many times; I am surprised at the genuine optimism in her voice. I want my reply to match her optimism. I should offer, for a change, an upbeat reply to match her fresh, morning mood. I check in with my body. I feel a stiffness that betrays my young age and a familiar pain in nearly all my muscles that if I didn't know better would suggest I had not slept the previous night but had instead been hoisting concrete for the last nine hours. Her expression changes from concern to anticipation. "Well?" she asks.

I reply, "Isn't rigor mortis supposed to set in *after* I die?"

"Kind of stiff today?" she asks, already knowing the answer.

I nod. There's no point even trying to describe or quantify the stiffness that has become as much a part of my morning routine as looking in the mirror or the pain that is at times incapacitating. But I am not discouraged because I know what will make me feel better...

Acknowledgments

Unlike other venues where individual people are thanked for their inspiration and perspiration, books offer the opportunity to thoroughly thank everyone without the risk of being interrupted with music, led off stage by a grinning model, or getting back to your seat and realizing you forgot to mention someone.

It makes the most sense to begin at the beginning, which for this book means thanking Jackie Boucher. It was her connections, creativity, and confidence that provided the spark that ignited this project. Thank you so much!

To the rest of my past and present colleagues at Health-Partners: your combined talents and personalities have created the most wonderful place to work and learn.

Many thanks are due to Betsy Thorpe at Wiley. After jumping into this project midstream, she's done an excellent job of providing wonderful feedback and edits. A hearty thank you is also due to Claire Huismann at Impressions Book and Journal Services.

I have been so blessed with supportive friends. There are so many of these jewels in my treasure chest that make my days shine and sparkle. Perhaps the most noticeable gem is my partner. She pushes me, loves me, and never fails to make me laugh a dozen times a day. My fibromyalgia has affected nearly every aspect of her life, and for her patience, persistence, and care I'm so grateful. Her intense loyalty and belief in self-improvement keep my fires lit. For this, and so much more, thank you, Schelly.

My parents, Larry and Olene Bigelow, are the keepers of a debt I can never repay. They made my early environment so full of unconditional love, which has been the most important and influential gift of my entire life. If you ever want to be inspired by a couple who overcame so much and still managed to give everything they had, get to know my parents.

The only other gift from them I treasure more than that love is that of my irreplaceable sister, Jill. I literally cannot imagine a moment in life without her nearby. Her priceless laugh, endless compassion, and loyal support have made life worth living.

My extended family, particularly my grandmothers, Margaret Hanson and Millie Bigelow, and my Aunt Ona and Uncle Vern have provided me with a connection to my past that, regretfully, I'm only now mature enough to fully appreciate.

No one manages fibromyalgia in a vacuum, and I'm no exception. In addition to my wonderful family, I would like to acknowledge the following people for their endless love and support: Julie Smith, Georgia Spiropoulos, James Haglund, Elizabeth "Bit" Turcotte, Hadas Tahir, Shane Deleers, Chris Enstad, Carol Nickel, Renee Robbins, Kira Camp, and Stan and Judy Sherr and their family. And a special thank you to the best massage therapist in the world, Ellen Zimmerman.

Introduction

Unless you have personally experienced the pain of fibromyalgia, there's no way to fully empathize with someone who has. The closest comparison I've found is how the survivor of a serious car accident feels 24 to 48 hours after the crash. It's as though every inch of your body has solidified like concrete. The constant pain makes the rest of the world fade into the background and uses every molecule of energy to accomplish only the bare essentials of daily life.

But, of course, you don't *look* sick. And you didn't just have an accident or other trauma that would allow both you and the rest of the world to explain or understand the pain. So you push yourself to get up every day and do what you can, despite being told that nothing is physically wrong with you, or that what *is* wrong with you, fibromyalgia, isn't a real condition.

The treatment for fibromyalgia can oftentimes seem as though it narrows our world even further. Extensive time and money is spent on varying medical treatments, books, and medications. Side effects and endless pain interrupt every aspect of life. Jobs are lost, and relationships suffer. Hope for a pain-free life evaporates along with the desire to keep trying one more thing to ease the pain.

But there may be one more thing worth trying. If you are like most people feeling their way through the facts and fictions of treating fibromyalgia, you have very likely missed something obvious: movement.

Chronic pain makes an increase in movement seem as likely as waking up tomorrow on a different planet. Usually this is because you either haven't tried it or because you've tried doing it incorrectly. Whether movement has come to mean something to avoid or something to endure, I promise you that there's room for you to feel better.

If you have fibromyalgia and want to have less pain, you need to move. This does not mean that you should exercise the way someone without fibromyalgia does. And it definitely does not mean your only option for exercise is in a warm-water pool. Don't settle for information that is not specific to fibromyalgia when it comes to activity and exercise.

This book is intended for people who have fibromyalgia but are still living with excessive pain and feel that the condition controls them, rather than feeling that they control the condition. It's for people who have never been able to create and maintain a routine of activity and exercise. It's especially for people who feel out of shape or overweight and struggle with chronic pain.

This book is not a resource for general information about fibromyalgia. There are wonderful books already available for that, several of which are listed at the end of this book. Each of them mentions the importance of activity and exercise, but to date, none of them have offered any in-depth information on how or whether to adapt traditional exercise recommendations to the condition of fibromyalgia. It is from the solid base of those books that this one begins.

My personal journey with fibromyalgia probably began in adolescence. I assumed that it was normal to wake up stiff and achey. Everyone in my family certainly did, and I was no exception. By the time I reached my early twenties, the pain had progressed to the point that I was starting to show up at the doctor's office with complaints of chronic pain, headaches, numbness in my hands, and other vague symptoms.

The resulting treatment was equally vague. I spent nearly two years in physical therapy that rarely helped and often left me feeling worse. Virtually every medical person I saw told me I must have some kind of injury and should rest until I felt better. One physical therapist explicitly banned me from exercise of any kind, and another encouraged it. One said to use heat, and another warned me to use only ice. One physician said my only option was surgery on my spine, and another said my last hope was to receive cortisone injections. One pain management program suggested I use visualizations, another suggested consulting a psychic. I read books that argued that I was causing the condition (which at this point didn't have a name) for a reason, and that all I needed to do was remove that reason and I would be healed. I spent years in psychotherapy sifting through some crippling issues, and although I felt stronger and healed emotionally, the physical pain persisted.

During these years and throughout my young adult life, I continued my professional training in psychology, health and fitness, teaching, and counseling. Although I was diagnosed with fibromyalgia in 1989, no one really taught me how to care for my condition, and my work suffered as a result. Chronic pain became so debilitating that doctors told me I'd have to quit my career and receive disability benefits. My entire life became about survival from day to day. I struggled to give quality care to my clients but knew my work was below my ability. I knew something had to change, and soon.

In my personal life, nearly every relationship suffered. I had no energy to socialize, and in the most severe stages of the pain, I had become unable to speak, smile, sing, or laugh without excruciating pain. With these parts of life gone, what was there left to live for? I couldn't answer that question, because even the hope of ever feeling better was gone.

Slowly, the medical knowledge about fibromyalgia grew. Slowly, I connected with people who knew what they were doing when they treated me. Slowly, I learned how to manage the pain and started to see it not as a curse but as a signal from my body. Slowly, I relearned how to exercise, relax, and eat in a way that made life feel normal again.

Perhaps a wonderful physician I recently met can sum up all the books, medical appointments, treatments, and pain. I was in Hawaii on vacation and was staying at a bed and breakfast on the big island. One of the owners was a traditional physician (M.D.) who had gone on for certification as a Doctor of Chinese Medicine. Over breakfast one morning, we began discussing fibromyalgia. Not one to mince words or beat around the bush, she said in a heavy Southern drawl, "Fibromyalgia ain't nuthin' but uptight." I had to think about this for a couple of weeks, but I gradually came to realize that she was right. People with fibromyalgia tend to respond to any stress with neuromuscular pain. If the sun's too bright, you get a headache. If you sit too long, you start to solidify in your seat. If you are upset about a conflict with another person, you feel muscular pain. The more pain you have, the more you respond with tension and pain. People may describe you as laid-back or easygoing, but if you have fibromyalgia, you can consider yourself an expert about being uptight. Movement is one of the most powerful ways to undo this process.

It *is* possible for you to feel better. It *is* possible for you to manage fibromyalgia, and it *will* require you to change. For me the choice was easy: if making changes would ease the pain, I would make the changes—any changes—I needed to. I hope you can make the same choice.

My work as a teacher, researcher, counselor, and behavior-change specialist has given me countless opportunities to work with people making changes for many reasons. Regardless of whether you want to lose weight, eat better, quit smoking, reduce your stress, manage a chronic condition, have less pain, leave a relationship, improve your communication skills, or do anything else, you will need to be willing to do things differently. If there were one thing I could give you, it would be the hope that those changes will be worthwhile. I extend that gift to you. Will you accept it?

CHAPTER 1

Concrete Lessons

If you have been diagnosed with fibromyalgia, you have probably been told repeatedly to exercise. If you are like most people, the word *exercise* immediately conjures up images of hard physical work, spending lots of time in a gym, and dealing with the low energy and pain that inevitably come after exercising. You may have been told that the only exercise you can do is in a heated pool, or possibly that there is nothing that can be done for fibromyalgia. If you are really motivated and assertive with your medical care, you may have had someone sit down with you and lay out a conventional exercise program. You may have found that when you try to exercise your pain gets *worse*, not better. Perhaps you feel so tired, sore, and stiff that exercising seems as likely as winning the lottery. It's not uncommon to feel discouraged, hopeless, and fed up with trying to exercise or get any relief from your pain.

Before you resign yourself to a life of constant pain and inactivity, ask yourself, "Has anyone told me *how* to use movement to ease my pain? Have I ever been given suggestions of how to use movement to care *specifically* for fibromyalgia?" If the answer is no, you're not alone. The average person diagnosed with fibromyalgia may not be given any guidance on how to use movement to relieve pain, and those told to exercise will often do so only to find the pain gets worse. If you have become very inactive, you may have gained weight and begun to experience other problems that make pain and immobility even worse, such as knee, foot, or back pain. You may feel you have no time to get more activity and are simply fated to a life with chronic pain. It's easy to understand how frustrated and exhausted you might feel. Whether you are an exercise veteran or consider changing TV channels a good work-out, there is hope!

By the time you finish reading this book you will know the following:

- The key to managing fibromyalgia
- Why traditional exercise programs are not for you
- How to determine which activities will cause you increased pain (and should be avoided) and which ones will reduce your pain
- The difference between physical activity and exercise
- How to know the difference between pain that's telling you to rest and pain that's telling you it's time to get moving
- How much movement and how much rest is enough
- How (and whether) to use muscle conditioning to decrease pain
- How to stretch properly to reduce pain
- How to communicate your needs to family members, coworkers, and health care providers

While you read this book, I'd like you to allow yourself the luxury of a new mind-set about your pain, body, and previous experience with exercise, activity, and movement. Whether you were very athletic as a child or the last one picked for teams in phys-ed class, put those self-concepts aside for now. They'll be there for you to pick up at the end of the book if you choose to do so. As you work through the ideas presented here, remain open to the possibility that your experience of pain and movement can be different. Imagine a door opening in your mind, letting fresh air into the stagnant room of chronic pain. Let's clear the air of some common misconceptions about fibromyalgia and pain and begin to rethink the options you have. If you are already sold on the idea of exercise and have no difficulty keeping an active lifestyle, feel free to jump ahead to the next chapter. But the rest of us will begin at a stoplight.

A Concrete Lesson

Imagine that you are standing at a stoplight waiting to cross the street. You hear a thundering sound approaching the intersection, and when you turn to look for the source of the sound, you see a giant truck pulling up and stopping in front of you. Upon closer inspection you notice that this is a cement truck. What's unique about a cement truck that makes it different from a truck that carries dirt? The back of the truck is moving, right? It's constantly moving and mixing its contents in a rounded barrel. Stop and think a moment. Why does a cement truck keep turning its contents? What would happen if the cement truck were to stop the constant mixing motion? It keeps turning because cement will stay soft as long as it keeps moving. But if it were to stop the rotation, the cement would solidify into concrete—rock solid and almost impossible to soften again.

The cement truck pulls away but leaves you with a special new insight: fibromyalgia causes your muscles to act like concrete. They require more movement than those of a regular body, and without that movement they will set and get hard and painful.

The most important key to managing muscles affected by fibromyalgia is to *keep them moving*. In case this key point may have missed you, let me restate it: The key to managing fibromyalgia is to keep your body moving, ideally in as gentle a manner as possible. There are other things to consider and utilize, such as medications, but by far the most important thing you can do, as well as the most effective form of pain relief, is to keep your body moving. Just as you can take a pain reliever (such as aspirin) for a headache, you can use movement to relieve pain.

Why Me?

Naturally, if you have fibromyalgia, you want to know *why*. Unfortunately, the list of what is known and generally accepted about fibromyalgia is small and rapidly changing. At this time, it's classified as a neuroendocrine condition. This means that fibro-myalgia seems to affect the way the body communicates pain to the brain and the systems that govern this communication and additional communication that occurs within your body. In the simplest of terms, you have a chemical imbalance that is setting off a cascade of symptoms in your body. You are probably all too aware of the various symptoms of fibromyalgia, and body pain is almost certainly right at the top of the list. Other common symptoms include tender, or trigger, points in a wide variety of locations on the body, as well as fatigue, stiffness, anxiety, and poor sleep.

Most people with fibromyalgia experience pain in their muscles. It has been shown that there are biological differences in the muscles of people with fibromyalgia, but it's thought that these differences are a result of the condition, not the cause. For example, there is usually less blood flow and hence less oxygen in muscles affected by fibromyalgia. There also seems to be a difference in how the muscles *respond* and the speed at which they heal.

Normal muscle tissue is soft when it's in a relaxed position. Relax your left arm, and reach over and feel the muscles just above the crease in the elbow. They should feel soft and spongy to the touch. When a normal muscle is moved gently (such as when you shop for groceries), the blood flow to the muscle increases and the oxygen level in the muscle increases. When finished with the job, the muscles rest again by returning to a soft, relaxed state. Any small tears in the muscle tissue are repaired and the muscles are restored to their prework level.

During intense exertion such as lifting weights, blood and oxygen levels increase as in the previous example, but this time the muscle fibers tear and break down considerably more. The body unaffected by fibromyalgia responds to this demand by rebuilding the muscle fibers stronger than they were before the exercise session. It's as though the body says, "If she's going to be doing *that* kind of work, I had better make her muscles stronger, so they're ready." The body adapts to the conditions that it's regularly exposed to, which is how exercise makes us stronger and why lack of care causes the body to decondition. When does the body do this adapting to exercise? When it's exercising? No. The body adapts during rest, partly during a certain stage of sleep, which will be discussed later.

Now reach up to your shoulder and walk your fingers in a couple of inches, so you are midway between your shoulder and neck. Push down gently. Feel the difference? If you are like many people with fibromyalgia, these muscles feel hard and rigid, and they lack the soft, pliable quality of healthy muscles. They may feel so hard and rigid you might think you are pressing on bone by mistake! They often have tender points that can be so painful that even gentle touch is uncomfortable. When you engage in mild motion such as unpacking groceries, any tiny tears in the tissue do not repair as readily, and the blood and oxygen levels are often below normal. As you finish your task the muscles get stiff and sore, making it less likely that you'll do more activity, which in turn causes more stiffness. If you try to do the weight lifting described in the previous paragraph, your muscles get tiny tears during the exercise, which is normal; however, they then fail to repair in the following 24 hours the way a normal muscle would. Your body tends to overreact to the whole experience and stiffens up with a combination of normal soreness after exercise and abnormal stiffness and pain due to the fibromyalgia.

Getting Your Z's

There's another crucial variable here, however, and that's the quality of your sleep. It's thought that a significant part of fibromyalgia is due to a lack of what's called *restorative sleep*. Restorative sleep is one of several stages of sleep, during which your body repairs damaged tissue (such as muscle), and people with fibromyalgia almost always miss this crucial stage. In fact, it's been found that if you take people without fibromyalgia, hook them up to monitors while they sleep, and then interrupt them every time they approach the restorative stage, they will develop symptoms very similar to those of fibromyalgia. It's easy to see how the lack of restorative sleep can lead to a vicious circle of unending pain; poor sleep causes more pain, pain causes poor sleep, and so on.

At this point, you might be asking yourself the chicken and the egg question. Does a sleep disorder cause fibromyalgia or does fibromyalgia cause a sleep disorder? The final answer to that question isn't known yet, but the good news for you is that the answer doesn't matter! Regardless of the cause and effect relationship of poor sleep and chronic pain, you can begin to intervene on either side of the problem and progress from there. There are several ways to increase the chances of getting enough restorative sleep, and there are ways to reduce pain and stiffness. I usually recommend that people begin to improve their sleep and then begin to manage any pain that has not been relieved by good sleep.

One of the best ways to ensure that you are getting restorative sleep is to use medications. The medications used for fibromyalgia are usually from the group of drugs known as antidepressants, which encourage restorative sleep. Unless you have depression in addition to fibromyalgia, you will usually take a lower dose than someone who is being treated for depression. Side effects are usually mild (such as a dry mouth), and virtually all side effects disappear after two weeks.

If after a few months on the medications you decide they're not helping, you can always stop taking them. Be sure to discuss how to do this with your doctor before discontinuing them. If you do it in the wrong way, you may feel worse than you did while taking them. Be patient and meticulous in how you take them. Together you and your doctor can determine the best place to start.

It's also important that you speak with your doctor to see if any other medications you are taking could be *interfering* with your restorative sleep. Many of the tranquilizing drugs, including alcohol, actually *reduce* the amount of restorative sleep you get, despite their main effect of making you sleepy. Because most people with fibromyalgia describe sleep problems, doctors often prescribe a mild sedative, unintentionally making the problem worse for you.

Other variables that can affect your sleep include:

- The quality and condition of your mattress
- The quality and condition of your pillow
- The temperature of your room
- The level of darkness
- The amount of distractions during the night, such as a partner who comes home late and wakes you, snores, or hogs the covers; or noise from children, pets, traffic, or neighbors that may disturb you
- Working late or overnight shifts
- Having irregular sleep/wake times

Most of the patients I've worked with sleep best while on medications, with a mattress on the soft side of firm, and in a very quiet, dark room. Supportive pillows and natural fiber sheets (such as all cotton) may also help. Of course, you may have different preferences. I'm asking you to think about what works best for you and to make those changes.

After all this talk about how incredibly important restorative sleep is, you might be wondering, "How will I know if I'm getting restorative sleep?" Great question. People who get restorative sleep:

- Wake up feeling rested and alert, not stiff, sore, and exhausted
- Dream nightly and often remember their dreams; do not have frequent nightmares
- Sleep through the night and do not wake up frequently

If you are starting to think you may have never had a good night's sleep, it's time to see your doctor to find out if you are a candidate for medication to help you sleep.

It's known that exercise will improve restorative sleep; however, I don't suggest that you begin using exercise to manage your sleep. You could actually make your pain worse by exercising and then failing to heal during the night. You need quality sleep first. You probably never thought you'd hear someone in the health professions telling you to not exercise, but if you have not been sleeping as you should for at least two weeks, that's exactly what I'm telling you to do. Don't exercise. Whether you are getting restorative sleep will determine what choices you have for activity and exercise. Invest some time into getting your body's natural healing process (sleep) up and running before you place more stress on it with exercise.

Getting Started

Once you are getting quality sleep on a regular basis, you are ready to start using movement to ease the remaining pain. I'm often asked if it's possible to use traditional exercise guidelines if you have fibromyalgia. The answer is no. There are three reasons why you should not use traditional exercise guidelines, even when you are sure you are getting restorative sleep.

First, there is a difference between activity and exercise, and it's critical that you understand the difference between the two to best care for fibromyalgia. If you don't get any activity but launch right into exercise, you'll be setting yourself up for days of pain. We'll discuss this in more depth later. To care for fibromyalgia you need as much activity as possible and gentle, moderate aerobic exercise. Regular exercise guidelines rarely mention activity. In addition, traditional exercise guidelines virtually never address your special needs. Even with the medications helping you get restorative sleep, you still need special guidelines for both of these important areas of movement.

Second, the medications don't alter the tendency for your muscles to stiffen during periods of inactivity or from movement that's too severe, so it is important that once you are getting good sleep, you have guidelines tailored to your condition. I've had clients tell me, "I'm in so much pain! I don't understand it because I'm taking my medications." Invariably after more probing, I find out they are sedentary most of the day, and when they do something physical, it's injurious. It's not fair to live as though you don't have fibromyalgia and then blame the medications for not doing their job. Getting restorative sleep is the first step. Then you need movement guidelines that are specific to fibromyalgia. This does not mean that some aspects of conventional exercise won't work just fine for you, but it's important to know what's fine and what isn't. That's what this book will help you do.

Lastly, your body will tend to heal and adapt to exercise more slowly than the body of someone without fibromyalgia, so the standard recommendations will often leave you in pain and without progress.

Changes to your activity and exercise should *always* be done one at a time, and I recommend that people make them in this order:

1. Make sure you are getting restorative sleep.
2. Get at least 60 minutes of activity per day, ideally 5 minutes of movement for every 30 minutes spent sedentary (the difference between activity and exercise will be discussed in Chapter 3).
3. Stretch at least five to seven times per week.
4. Do gentle aerobic exercise at least five to seven times per week.
5. Do muscle conditioning two to three times per week.

If this sounds overwhelming right now, relax. You don't *have* to do all of it. You don't have to do *any* of it. This is simply the order you should use for best pain relief. If you're still waking up feeling like the earth's gravitational pull suddenly got stronger during the night, you need to focus on the first item. Don't try to skip around in the list. Work through the sequence.

We'll be discussing fatigue further later on, but it is important to mention it here as well. One of the main symptoms of fibromyalgia is fatigue, and this is especially true if you are not getting restorative sleep. This can be a major problem because the main thing that helps ease the pain of fibromyalgia is movement, which takes some effort and energy, especially in the beginning. Low energy and low levels of activity feed off each other and contribute to pain.

Managing fibromyalgia successfully will require some effort on your part. You do not *have* to exercise or even increase your level of activity. You have a choice. If you prefer to live with a higher pain level (and the other health risks associated with an inactive life), that may be a valid choice for you right now. There are trade-offs for every choice you make in life, and managing your fibromyalgia is no different. The advantage of a sedentary life is that no effort is spent finding ways to be gently active. The downside is a life with more pain, fatigue, and limits. By choosing less pain, you will be spending more energy and time on staying active. Remember the gift to yourself of staying open-minded about your pain, movement, and your body, and consider starting with a small change.

Anytime we decide to make a change in our lives it requires a certain amount of energy and planning. We need to be *ready* to change. One person reading this book may be making plans to get more activity in her life, while another might only be considering it. Still another person might be very active and exercising already, but interested in making modifications.

I recently worked with one young woman who reminded me of how important it is to be honest with yourself about change. She had been diagnosed with fibromyalgia many years earlier but had not taken an active role in caring for it. One questionnaire asked her what her weekly goals were for aerobic exercise. When I spoke with her later, she said that she thought the questions about exercise were useless and stupid. I suggested we talk about why she felt that way. She said, "Well, I knew the right answer was three to four times a week, so I put that. But that is completely unrealistic for my life right now. This whole section was useless to me." I asked her if it was possible that the reason it felt useless to her was because she didn't really consider what *her* answer was, but rather put in what she thought was the right answer. She considered this, and I encouraged her to rethink the question and come up with something that *would* be realistic for her life. In doing this, she decided that an honest answer was that taking short walks once or twice a week was possible, even enjoyable, for her, and would be significantly more exercise than she was currently getting. Try to use this perspective when you are thinking about your responses. It takes courage to consider any change, and even more courage when chronic pain is involved. The hope of less pain motivates us all.

In Review

Movement is an indispensable part of keeping your body from feeling as though it's made of cement.

Quality sleep is a foundation in treating fibromyalgia and must be in place before you attempt any exercise. Medications can be an indispensable way of improving your sleep and treating fibromyalgia. Do not attempt any exercises outlined in this book until you and your doctor are sure quality sleep is firmly in place.

There is hope! Most people who follow the guidelines in this book will have significantly less pain, depression, and anxiety; will often lose weight (if necessary); and will improve their overall health.

Making changes takes courage and honesty with yourself but is well worth the effort.

CHAPTER 2

Getting Motivated

When I ask my patients to name their primary barrier to movement, I hear unanimously, "Motivation. Help me get motivated!" I even had one woman describe her fondest wish to me. She said, "Stacie, why can't they come up with a machine that will move my arms and legs *for* me?" I remember thinking that she had a long way to go before she understood motivation. I've learned that what people are really saying is, "Make me *want* to do this!" What about you? Have you ever felt a lack of motivation to do activity or exercise?

Over the years, I've found some helpful ways to get out of a chronic case of low motivation. But be forewarned; this is not about me psyching you up to the point that you can hardly wait to go out and train for a marathon. It's also not about me berating you long enough that you go out and take a walk but feel as though you've been forced to go. And in case you believe motivation comes from hating yourself enough to do something about your miserable self, you may want to check yourself in for deprogramming. None of this is motivation.

Let me ask you something. Whatever you do for work, whether it's working for pay, managing a household, or volunteer work, how many days a week do you jump out of bed and joyfully get ready, salivating at the thought of spending the day (or night) doing your work? Not every day? So there are some days you don't want to work? What do you do about that feeling? Do you call in and say, "You know, I just don't feel like coming in today. I'm afraid I'm going to have to wait until I feel like it"? Of course not. You get dressed, go to work, and make the best of it. You *do* have the ability to do things you don't want to do. It's part of being an adult and taking responsibility for yourself.

You might say, "I'd get fired if I didn't show up every time I didn't feel like going." True, but doesn't work (or maintaining a household, or raising kids) provide you with benefits you can't get anywhere else? Isn't it true that the consequences of not working are greater than the cost of going to work, even when you don't feel like it?

The reality is that you *choose* to go to work. You don't *have* to go. You choose to go because you need what work gives you: money, benefits, personal satisfaction, a better life for you and your family, and a host of other things. Exercise is no different.

When people tell me that they just don't feel like exercising, I ask them, "Why do you have to feel like doing it?" I agree it helps, but it's not required. And it externalizes your responsibility for making the choice to move or to sit. It implies that you are a victim to yourself, that if only this low level of motivation didn't burden you, you'd be out there romping around like a six-year-old child. Motivation follows action, not the other way around. If you wait until you feel like doing everything, very little will get done. And you'll be in a lot of pain. Part of motivation is simply allowing yourself to do something you might not feel like doing at the moment, in the name of a payoff.

I can't tell you how many times I've heard people complain relentlessly about how movement takes too much time, isn't fun, feels like work, and so on. There are endless ways to make movement fun, enjoyable, and less painful. Figure out how and do it.

If you're not going to do it, own that choice and leave it at that. Rather than saying, "I really should, but I don't want to," you can just say, "I'm not going to exercise today, and I accept that I might be stiff and sore later on because of it." That's all there is to it. Don't make it bigger than it is.

Another reason for low motivation is boredom. I can hear it in the voices of my patients: "I don't know what's wrong with me. I just can't make myself get on that treadmill." Or, "I can't stand the thought of that gym." I wonder why their motivation is low. Invariably when I ask them if they *like* using the treadmill or going to the gym, they say, "Ugh, no! I hate it! But I have to exercise, don't I?"

No, you don't *have* to exercise. You can choose not to. But if you *want* to exercise, you deserve to like what you are doing. If a root canal sounds more tolerable than what you have planned for movement, it's time to come up with another plan.

At this point, I ask people what they like to do. They start to perk up right away. They start to sound playful and bouncy as they describe wrestling with their kids, playing at the park with their dog, hiking on wooded trails, and gardening. Then, after finally finding their elusive motivation, they proceed to talk themselves right out of it again. "But that's not exercise," they say. Of course it is! Now, if you're training for the Olympics, it's not exercise, but for almost everyone else it is. At the very least it counts as activity. And it certainly helps fibromyalgia! Don't deny yourself the joy of movement.

The fabulous fitness expert Covert Bailey asks his audiences how many of them stay on an exercise bike one second after the timer bell rings. No one raises his or her hand. But how many of us have gone just a little longer on a walk just because it was a beautiful evening and we felt so wonderful? Almost everyone I know can say yes to that. In addition to the fact that becoming more fit will improve almost every aspect of your life, one thing is certain: you won't do what you don't enjoy. So be sure you find, and do, what you love.

Every once in a while I have a tough-nut client who, at this point in the conversation, will say, "There's nothing I like to do." "Fine," I say, "then just sit there and hurt." If you are more committed to your pain than to your recovery, there's nothing I, or anyone else, can do for you.

The "I'll do it later" answer to low motivation is like contributing to a slow death. Many people don't realize this, but I want to let you in on a secret. It's possible for your health to be too far gone for you to be *able* to do it later. You don't believe me? Then learn from my patients. I have several patients who are in their fifties or older, have fibromyalgia, are very overweight, and have developed severe joint pain. One woman desperately needs a hip replacement but can't have the surgery until she loses 50 pounds. She's let herself go for so long that she can't exercise until the hip is replaced. No exercise, no weight loss. No weight loss, no surgery. No surgery, no exercise. There's a very good chance she'll spend the remaining years of her life in continuous pain, over-weight, and miserable. The one thing she can still do is gentle movement in a pool. Do you know what she says when I ask her if she's gone to the pool? "I'll get to it sometime. I just don't have the motivation." If you wait too long, it might be too late.

In Review

It's not necessary to feel like exercising in order to do it.

It's possible for it to be too late to exercise later.

Take responsibility for your decision to either exercise or not and consciously accept the pros and cons of your choice.

CHAPTER 3

Keep It Moving!

If you were going to read just one chapter of this book, it should be this one. If you do only one type of movement to care for your fibromyalgia, it should be activity.

What is activity, exactly? Activity and exercise once meant the same thing. Leading an active lifestyle meant jogging several times a week, working out at a gym, and stopping only to sleep. These definitions have changed! There's an important distinction between activity and exercise, and the recommended levels for each are different for people with fibromyalgia than for people without.

Think for a moment about your life and all the things that you do that involve movement, but don't count any structured exercise you may be doing. Do you go grocery shopping? Do you run errands on the weekend? Does your job involve walking around? Do you have young kids? If so, you undoubtedly move quite a bit to care for them. Are you in the middle of redecorating a room? Does doing the laundry involve going up or down stairs?

These actions are all examples of activity, and the general rule for activity is the more the better. There are some exceptions to this, and we'll cover those later. For now, just think through your days and get a feel for the types of things you do that keep you moving.

Activity is the foundation of managing fibromyalgia. It is most effective when done along with mild, regular aerobic exercise. But activity without exercise is better than exercise without activity. Here's an example:

Joanne is 67 and retired. Her fibromyalgia was diagnosed when she was 52. She worked as a school nurse for 40 years and now enjoys time at home with her husband and visits with her grandchildren. Her favorite pastimes are crocheting and reading. She lives in a condominium, so there is no yard work for her to do. She began thinking she should get some exercise (her doctor told her it would help the fibromyalgia pain), so three times a week she either goes for a walk (weather permitting) or uses a treadmill, which she bought at a garage sale about a year ago. She normally walks for about 30 minutes, although she often has too much pain and stiffness, which causes her to skip the exercise.

Emily is 49 and runs a housecleaning business. She often works 10-hour days, which mainly involves cleaning several houses a day. Her fibromyalgia was diagnosed in her early thirties when she was put on bed rest for the last month of her pregnancy. Until then she had only mild pain and occasional headaches when she felt she had overdone it at work. She has never exercised regularly because she usually feels too tired at the end of the day to even think about it.

There are 10,080 minutes in a week. Joanne, on a good week, moves her body for less than 60 of those minutes (remember activity and exercise are counted separately) and gets occasional movement minutes from exercise. Most of her activity comes in very brief bursts, such as taking a shower, making a meal, or walking around the house.

Emily, on the other hand, gets about 3,000 minutes of activity a week just from working five days, and that's not counting her grocery shopping, gardening, caring for her kids, and all the other chores of caring for herself and her family. She doesn't exercise, but she is almost always in motion. In fact, until she *stopped* moving, she never even knew she had fibromyalgia! She was already doing such a good job of managing it (without knowing she had it) that she had virtually no symptoms.

Now that you know (and hopefully understand) that the best way to ease pain from fibromyalgia is to move as often and as gently as possible, who is doing the best job? Who has the best level of pain? If you were to talk to them, Joanne might say she is exercising but is still having debilitating pain. Emily may feel that she should be exercising, but her pain level is in good control. Again, this is not to say that exercise is not important or to underestimate the dramatic effect that aerobic exercise has on your health, but from the perspective of pain management for fibromyalgia, activity is the most important. Let's look at the lives of two other people with fibromyalgia.

Mary got her diagnosis of fibromyalgia in her early thirties after spending two years in physical therapy and seeing many doctors. She actually felt grateful for the diagnosis because her symptoms finally made sense and she could start taking some action to help her pain. Her doctor and physical therapist told her that exercise would help her pain level, and she decided to dust off some of her old exercise videotapes she had purchased to help her lose weight after graduating from college. She remembered that she always had headaches when she used them, which she attributed to the stress she was under with her first job out of college. The first time she used the tape was a Saturday morning while her husband took the kids to the zoo. As her body warmed up during the workout, she noticed her pain level got better, and by the end of the workout, she felt euphoric. "There's hope!" she thought. Later that night, as she was preparing dinner, she noticed a headache starting in the back of her neck and shoulders, which grew in intensity until she went to bed early that night. She awoke the next morning feeling very stiff and sore. She spent most of Sunday resting and reading and eventually took a nap. In the late afternoon, still feeling like she had been hit by a train, she decided she would try the aerobic dance tape again. "If it worked yesterday, it'll work today," she thought.

The second time through the tape wasn't as good as the first. As the instructor took her through the first dance sequence, she could feel the muscles in her upper body spasming into tight knots. After 15 minutes of the tape, she couldn't stand the pain anymore and went to lie down. She thought to herself, "I don't understand why I'm getting these headaches all of a sudden. I'm not under a lot of stress right now."

She slept on and off through the night and at 2 A.M. had finally resorted to taking a muscle relaxant her doctor had prescribed before her fibromyalgia was diagnosed. She awoke Monday morning with an excruciating headache and called in sick to work. Although she was able to work on Tuesday, it was several days before her pain level was low enough that she could even think about exercising again, but somehow the tape didn't sound so interesting anymore. She felt discouraged and hopeless that anything would help the pain of fibromyalgia, and she gave up on using exercise to manage it.

When she met with her doctor six months later to see how she was doing, she told him, "Exercise makes my fibromyalgia pain worse. Nothing seems to help."

Pat had always admired herself for not taking any medications. She believed that doctors always want to over-medicate their patients, and she had a personal experience with this that nearly killed her. She preferred using other remedies, such as homeopathy or herbs. When she was diagnosed with fibromyalgia, she declined her doctor's suggestion of using Elavil to help her restorative sleep and decided to try homeopathy. After two months of homeopathic treatment, using several remedies, although she felt more rested in the morning, the stiffness had not improved. She talked with her homeopathic practitioner about taking medications and decided to try a three-month experiment in conjunction with the homeopathy. After the first week she nearly gave up; she had no improvement in the stiffness and the side effect of a dry mouth. Both of her caregivers encour-

aged her to give it the full three months and reminded her if it wasn't working she could easily go off of the medications with no ill effects.

After three weeks, she woke up without feeling like she had been through a car accident the previous day! The dry mouth had passed about a week before, but this was the first time she had noticeably less stiffness. This allowed her to feel good enough to increase her activity and exercise levels, which in turn helped her balance her system through a healthy lifestyle. Although she still prefers not to take medications, she also understands that sometimes it is necessary for her health to take them carefully, and that it's also hard on her body to be missing a crucial stage of sleep.

In Mary's situation, she started to exercise without being active. In addition, she began with a type of exercise that overworked the muscles most affected by her fibromyalgia. She didn't understand that although exercise helps fibromyalgia, not just *any* exercise helps: first there needs to be a solid foundation of activity.

How Active Are You?

If you are very out of shape and plunge into an exercise program, odds are that, 48 hours after your first workout, when you're sore, you'll restrict your activity level, thinking it will help you recover from your exercise session. But the lack of activity will cause your muscles to set up like concrete faster than you can say, "Please get me some ibuprofen." A far more successful approach for someone who has not been exercising regularly is to start by assessing how much activity you are currently getting.

Stop and think about your typical week. Mentally tally up all the activity minutes you get in a normal day and write this amount down. If you have no idea how much activity you get in a day (and most people don't), you may want to consider investing a few days finding out. The least expensive and easiest way to do this is to carry a small notepad and a pencil with you and record the number of minutes you spend in movement. When you do this, do not count minutes spent doing intentional exercise (such as walking for 30 minutes or swimming for 45 minutes). *Do* include the time spent shopping, doing yard work, making the bed, walking to and from your car or bus stop, walking to the cafeteria from your desk, and doing anything else that's not sedentary. Typing or using a computer does not count as activity. Watching TV, even if you get up to change the channels, doesn't count either. A good rule of thumb is to count anything that uses your legs to move you for longer than one minute. You don't have to make this rocket science. If you want to estimate the number of minutes you walk around the office or care for your child, that's fine. Whatever works for you. Just try to get a general idea of what a typical day and week are for you. If you have a different schedule on workdays versus nonwork days, try to get a sample of at least one of each type of day. If you are about to leave on vacation for a week, there's not much point in tracking your activity level while you're gone because it won't be typical (although you should try to be as active as possible while you are gone).

Once you have a general idea of how many minutes of activity you get, you can start thinking about whether you are getting enough.

How Much Is Enough?

For a person without fibromyalgia, the recommendation is to accumulate at least 30 minutes of activity during the day, most days of the week. This is a minimum amount, and more is better.

For someone with fibromyalgia, the recommendation I use is at least twice that amount, or 60 minutes accumulated during the day, every day of the week. Again, more is better. The ideal for pain control is 5 minutes of movement for every 30 minutes of nonmovement.

In working over the years with patients (both with fibromyalgia and without), I have received several reactions to these guidelines. Most stay-at-home moms exclaim, "I've done 60 minutes of activity before 10 A.M.!" And they have. Others have always considered themselves inactive, but once they add up walking to and from their car or bus stop, taking care of the yard, doing laundry, grocery shopping, and so on, they realize they have very active lives, even if they aren't exercising regularly. Still others add up their minutes and realize they have (very effectively) removed all traces of activity from their life by making things as convenient and efficient as possible.

One example of this is provided by Julie, a woman I worked with about a year ago. Julie worked at a desk job, had no kids, and lived on a ground-floor apartment. Her typical day included her morning routine of eating breakfast, taking a bath, and reading the paper, driving to work, sitting all day in front of a computer, driving home, and sitting most evenings while she read or watched TV until she went to bed. When she got together with friends or went on a date, the plans usually included something sedentary: going out to eat, watching a movie, or playing board games. When she walked to her office building from her car and back again, she got a couple minutes of activity, although she always tried to find the closest parking space to the entrance. She usually brought her lunch to work and ate at her desk, so there was no need to walk to the cafeteria or even back to her closely parked car to go out for lunch. Julie had become an expert at inactivity! Not surprisingly, she had gained weight and felt her energy level was so low that even the process of grocery shopping drained any last bit of energy she had. She needed to start small and not try to exercise right away. After assessing her day, we discussed simple ways to begin increasing her activity level. I'll give you the same guidelines I gave Julie to easily increase your activity. When you're shooting for extra minutes, every minute counts. Here are some tips:

Simple Ways to Increase Activity

- Make daily tasks a little less convenient. This is probably one of the most effective ways of getting more activity, especially if you have a busy life. Park as far as you reasonably can from your destination rather than searching for the closest spot. Go to the water fountain or bathroom that is farthest from your desk at work. Take the stairs instead of the elevator or the escalator. Take the longer route to the store in the mall you're heading for. Walk to the mailbox a couple of blocks away instead of dropping your mail in the closest one. Do you ride the bus? Get off a couple of stops early. Wash your car by hand instead of driving through the car wash. (Be creative! Every extra minute spent in motion can mean less pain. You don't have to do everything in your life less conveniently; pick the things that are the easiest for you to realistically do).

- When is the least-active part of your day? Do you come home from work and lie around until you go to bed? Do you sit at work all day, limiting your movement to your fingers at the keyboard? These are the times where you can really make a difference in your pain level. Move!

- Do the more active chores at home. If standing at the sink doing dishes hurts your neck, and someone else does all the active chores, make a trade! Vacuuming, dusting, mowing the lawn, gardening, and anything else that keeps you gently moving will help.

- Learn to notice opportunities for brief movement. If you put your dinner into the microwave to defrost for 10 minutes, think, "I've got 10 minutes to walk around the block." If a friend calls to say she'll pick you up to go to a movie in 45 minutes, you can realize, "Sitting in a movie for two hours is sure to generate some pain, but I've got 45 minutes now. I think I'll take a walk for 15 minutes so I have less pain after the movie."

- Minimize long periods of sitting. When you plan a day or someone suggests an activity, think about it from a pain-management perspective. If on a rainy

Saturday morning you are planning to settle in for a long day of reading, stop and think if it's worth the trade-off of having more pain for the next day or two. It may sound crazy, but there will be times you will say yes to activities knowing full well that you're going to hurt because of it. But you can work some activity into your day to minimize this. If you want to read all day, you can take breaks to take a walk, vacuum the house, or do some stretching. If you are planning a road trip in the car, plan frequent stops to move around and stretch. When you know you'll be sitting for a long period, a little alarm bell should go off inside your head, along with the image of that cement truck from Chapter 1.

You can follow these guidelines whether or not you are on medications to help you sleep at night. This kind of movement is designed to keep your muscles from hardening while minimizing the risk of triggering more pain. Keep it gentle, and you'll be fine. You can listen to your body for clues. If you try to play tennis on Monday, and on Tuesday you need a crane to get out of bed, then you know to store your tennis racket. You may find that an activity that's totally intolerable now might be fine later as you increase your fitness. There will be a fair amount of trial and error as you learn to manage your pain. The zone you're aiming for contains a wide variety of activities that ease pain and don't trigger lots of pain later on. If you wait until you have no pain to begin becoming more active, then you've missed the whole point of this chapter.

As is true for any change you make, these changes will feel awkward and unnatural for about a month, and then they'll feel normal. Of course, having less pain will be a significant reward to help keep you going.

Don't make the mistake of underestimating the impact more activity can have on your life. You can feel the results of increasing your activity right away, oftentimes within minutes. In time, pain associated with fibromyalgia can be a signal to get up and move for a few minutes, much the way other pain is a signal to take a pain-relieving medication.

And That's Not All

In addition to providing pain relief, activity burns calories, which is important for a variety of reasons. Burning calories is important if you are trying to lose weight, and activity will help. A friend of mine, an exercise physiologist, recently shared some interesting facts with me. He said that the average 175-pound person would lose 6 pounds a year just by walking up and down two flights of stairs a day instead of taking the elevator, if all other aspects of eating and exercise were held constant. He also said that the average person with an active daily life (taking care of small children all day, or having a full-time job with lots of movement, such as nursing) burns about 3.5 calories per minute. Compare this to the sedentary person (such as one who has a desk job) who burns about 2 calories per minute. Do you think 1.5 calories per minute doesn't make a difference? Think again. At the end of one year, these 1.5 calories per minute will add up to 170,000 calories, which is equal to nearly 50 pounds of fat. Anyone who's had an active job and then gets a desk job has almost certainly noticed the difference this makes.

Activity also has a huge impact on the number of calories you burn in a day. How many activity calories do you think you burn in a day? Not sure? The number of calories you burn in one day depends on how much you weigh and how much muscle you have. But even without this information, you can still see what a difference activity makes.

Let's say you are single with no children, have a desk job, and drive to work. You spend your lunch hour eating with coworkers and your evenings watching TV. The total calories burned through activity are going to be about 100. That's it. You'll burn a few taking a shower, getting dressed, walking around your

office, and making dinner, but most of the time your body is idle.
You've burned more than 100 calories for the day from all the
other functions your body does, such as pumping blood, digest-
ing food, and maintaining your body temperature. But your calories coming from activity will be very low. Even if you exercise
that day, you'll burn only another couple hundred calories for the
whole day, depending on how long you exercise for.

Now let's imagine that you get a different job. Now you're a
nurse with small kids and an active partner. You're up at 5:30 to
get the kids ready for school. Because the kids need breakfast,
help getting dressed, and finding lost schoolbooks, the only time
you sit down is to put on your shoes. Because you work at a large
hospital, you have a significant walk to get to your station from
the parking ramp, and once you are there you never stop moving. You are constantly going from patient to patient providing
care, getting supplies, answering the phone, and helping other
staff. After working an 8-hour shift and picking up groceries,
you meet your kids at home for playtime, dinner, and homework. After everyone is in bed, you unwind with gentle yoga
stretching before bed.

In this scenario, you would have likely burned *2,000* calories
from activity! All the calories burned from other body functions
(which, incidentally, is a full 75% of your calorie burning) is *in
addition* to this! Any exercise you do is also in addition to this!
There's no question that this is a large amount of activity, but
even if you do only half of this, you are still burning up to 10
times the amount of calories from activity than if you are sedentary all day. Adding activity to your day allows you to burn 2,500
to 3,500 or more calories per day; without activity, you only burn
1,500. Whatever you do, don't underestimate the value of getting
lots of activity.

Calorie Counters and Pedometers

Would you like a closer estimate of how many calories
you burn in a day? A motion-sensitive device that can

tell you is available, and it's only the size of a personal pager. It's worn on the waist of your clothing, and after you program in your height, weight, and gender, it will count calories burned through activity as well as total calories burned during the day. It can provide an indispensable source of feedback about both your health and the pain of fibromyalgia because activity can dramatically help the pain. There are a couple of brands of calorie monitors, and you can check with a local fitness-equipment retailer for help finding one. They usually cost between $80 and $100.

A less-expensive gadget is a pedometer. These measure the number of steps you get in a day. This information can be converted to calories, but it's just as effective if you aim to get at least 10,000 steps a day. It may sound like a lot, but it really isn't!

In Review

Activity plays a crucial role in managing the pain of fibromyalgia.

Activity is any movement you do that is less intense than aerobic exercise or is done for less than 15 minutes.

For the best pain relief, get at least 5 minutes of activity for every 30 minutes spent sedentary.

There are almost limitless ways to increase the amount of activity you get in a day. Know how much you are currently getting and begin making changes to increase this.

In caring for fibromyalgia, activity without exercise is better than exercise without activity.

CHAPTER 4

Flexible Bodies Have Less Pain

On a typical day, do you feel more like a rubber band or a block of cement? Does it seem that *flexible* is a word that applies only to other people? When you hear the word *yoga*, does it immediately conjure up images of people twisted up like pretzels? If you already stretch, do you rush through the process in less than five minutes?

If your answers are less than encouraging, take heart. You have something to gain from this chapter.

Flexibility is one of the three essentials for fitness (along with aerobic exercise and muscle conditioning) and pain control. But stretching is often in the shadow of aerobic exercise, with little information available on its benefits or how to stretch most effectively.

Flexibility is crucial for health as well as optimal pain control. In other words, if you want less pain, you will need to stretch. And you will need to stretch correctly to get the most pain relief.

Stretching Might Feel Better Than You Think

Stretching, when done right, feels good. It's calming, centering, and connecting. It doesn't have to cost anything, has almost immediate benefits, and can be done anywhere. And, unlike aerobic exercise and muscle conditioning, you can stretch anytime regardless of how well you are sleeping. Do you still doubt the benefits? Are you saying to yourself, "Stacie, I've been stretching for years and it never does everything you claim it does?" If you're feeling reluctant to invest some more time in stretching, read on.

I'd like you to picture an elderly woman walking across the room. What's her posture like? What kind of steps does she take? If you were to ask her to bend over and touch her toes, how far would she be able to reach? Do you think all of this restricted movement is just old age? Guess again! Although certainly some of her cautious movements are related to advanced age, the majority are caused from not maintaining normal flexibility with stretching. Even without fibromyalgia, much of the back and neck pain people experience is a direct result of poor flexibility. For the people who do take the time to stretch, most do it incorrectly and either get minimal benefits or may even hurt themselves while stretching.

If you'd like to avoid being a pain-bound, tight, inflexible person, then stretching can help you. Your ability to stretch is only partially affected by your genetic makeup. Although this can account for some differences between people, I have no doubt that stretching can improve your flexibility and reduce your pain.

Of course, you'll need to do it right. Keep it simple, and don't panic as you learn (or relearn) to stretch. Remember the goal is to have less pain. Allow yourself some time and maybe to even enjoy the process.

What Exactly Is Stretching?

Stretching can mean everything from a few shoulder rolls after sitting at a desk for too long to becoming a yoga master. So let's start by defining what will help the pain. I will provide you with some pictures of helpful stretches, but don't feel limited to those. There are as many ways to stretch as there are ways to move. I will also provide plenty of advice about stretching, and I hope you'll consider some of it and see what stretching can do for you and the pain.

By this point I'm hoping you are at least curious to see what all the fuss is about and are open to thinking about stretching in a new way. Let's lay some ground rules. For each of the following points, I've included a visual image called *Picture This* to help convey the meaning. You may find it helpful to use this image while you stretch.

Stretching is gentle. At no time should you feel pain or as though you're going to break in half if you stretch one more inch. Although this is true for everyone, it's especially true for people with fibromyalgia. If you stretch aggressively, you run the risk of increasing the pain, not reducing it.

Picture This:

You are dressing a newborn baby. You move the baby's arms and legs gently into the sleeves and legs, and carefully put the socks and shoes on the baby's feet.

It's also very important that you stretch slowly. You will need to be quietly connected to your body so that you can hear the signals to stretch further, hold a position, and release. If you move directly into the full stretch, release abruptly, and then launch into the next position, you will miss nearly all the benefits of stretching. Move into each position slowly and hold it for at least 20 seconds while you breathe deeply. When you are ready to release, gently come out of the pose before beginning the next. You will find that some poses flow wonderfully from one to another to make a slow, relaxing dance. If you have only five minutes to stretch, it's better to do two or three stretches slowly than to rush through ten.

Picture This:

Your body has been reprogrammed to move in slow motion, and you have all the time in the world.

It will help if you can remain calm while you stretch. If you are starting to lose your balance, listening for the doorbell, or making grocery lists in your head, you won't be calm. If you are really paying attention to your body and breathing, remaining calm and focused will be easy.

Picture This:

You are a willow tree calmly growing next to a lake. You have nothing to fear and nothing to worry about.

Lastly, when you stretch you should feel in control of your body. I do not mean that you should force yourself into a painful stretch, but that you are thoughtfully choosing each step in the process. If you feel like you are flailing all over the place and making it up as you go, you are not stretching with control. Your moves should be deliberate.

Picture This:

You are crossing a stream by stepping on rocks. You choose the next rock to step on only after some consideration.

Here is a review of stretching:

- Gentle—like dressing a baby
- Slow—like moving in slow motion
- Calm—like a willow tree by a lake
- Controlled—like crossing a stream on stones

Keeping these ideas in mind (and body) will help you get all the benefits that stretching has to offer.

Although stretching takes some mild effort, you want to avoid working at stretching. If you put too much effort into stretching, you might finish feeling *more* tense than when you started. To help you capture this balance between effort and no effort, remember to do the following.

Relax. As you move into each stretch, release any tension in the rest of your body. If you've been in constant pain for a long time, this may be difficult. Do the best you can. Concentrate on the area of your body you are stretching and let go of the rest.

Breathe normally. You should be inhaling and exhaling comfortably, and under no circumstances should you hold your breath. This decreases the amount of oxygen in your muscles and creates more muscle tension.

Stretch gently and comfortably. If you were to rate yourself on a scale of 1 to 10 (with 10 being the most intense), you should be around a 4 or 5. Level 1 would be reaching for an object near you and 10 would be intense straining. At 4 or 5, the stretch should feel good.

Hold the position for at least 20 seconds. This is why it's so important to not stretch beyond what is comfortable. Rather than counting in your head (which can keep you too focused on finishing the stretch), count your breaths. If you are relaxed, you will be breathing slowly and easily, with roughly eight seconds or more elapsing from the start to the finish of the breath. If you count four or five of these breaths, you'll be ready to move to the next stretch. Never bounce when you stretch; this increases your chance of injury. Simply hold the position. If you feel at all uncomfortable or tense, release the stretch slightly until you can hold it easily for 20 to 30 seconds. I've also included some stretches that can be held for 5 to 10 minutes, and those are noted in the description below the picture.

Make slow transitions into and out of each stretch. Try to keep your mind calm during the stretch while you move into the next one. Move slowly, breathe normally, and place your body carefully.

Be willing to modify stretches if necessary. Trying to stretch beyond what is comfortable won't help you relax or ease pain.

Modifying stretches is easy—simply don't stretch as far. When you modify a stretch, you are still stretching correctly and still receiving all of the benefits.

Unless you have some other injury or illness, there are no stretches you can't do if you follow the guidelines above.

Many people are familiar with traditional, or athletic, stretches, but there are many others. On the following pages are some good stretches that target parts of the body often affected by fibromyalgia, but they are by no means the only stretches you can do. While they can be used alone, it is best to use them along with other stretches.

Remember to breathe normally, go slowly, and move gently. If you have several minutes to devote to stretching, it helps to be in loose-fitting, comfortable clothing. If you are taking a short break during your day, you may want to undo the top button along your waist or remove anything especially restrictive. If neither of these options is possible, simply do what's comfortable.

Invariably, very flexible people teach stretching. And inevitably the participants in the class try to emulate the instructor and get frustrated. Here's my tip for keeping this from happening to you. Think of the demonstrated stretch as the speed limit. Speed limits are set as the maximum speed possible under the best of conditions. When there is rain, ice, construction, darkness, or traffic, you are expected to adjust your speed to the conditions. Stretching is exactly the same. The demonstrated stretch usually represents the maximum stretch possible, and you will need to modify it for your physical condition. Yes, the instructor is more flexible than you are, and you can't stretch as far as you might like to. None of this matters. To get the benefits, you need to adjust what is demonstrated to the current condition of your body. To do otherwise is like trying to speed on a freeway clogged with traffic and icy roads: sooner or later it's going to cause an accident. Don't make this mistake with your body. You already have enough pain; don't cause yourself more.

In the following box is a script that can be read to you by a helper while you stretch. If you do not live with someone who will do this for you, see if there's someone else in your life who will. You might even want to record it for yourself so you can play it back while you stretch. It will help make the stretching as beneficial as possible. I also encourage you to stretch while listening to soothing music. Music has a profound impact on our bodies, and it can tremendously enhance the benefits of stretching.

Stretching Script

Stand comfortably. Begin with a slow, deep breath. Feel the breath begin to relax and calm your muscles. Take another slow, deep breath. Feel the oxygen circulating to tight muscles and imagine it dissolving tight knots and relaxing pressure points. Repeat to yourself quietly: all is well... all is well... all is well. Take one more slow deep breath. As you exhale, imagine your muscles feeling warm and fluid.

Move into the first stretch you want to do slowly, keeping your calm state of mind. Continue to breathe normally. Stretch into position gently, stopping before you feel discomfort. Hold and breathe normally. Continue to hold, and with each exhalation imagine air dissolving any tightness. As the tightness releases, repeat quietly to yourself: all is well... all is well... all is well... After 5 to 10 breaths in this manner, gently release the stretch back to a resting position. Keep your mind calm and continue to breathe. Slowly release the stretch and move into the next position. Stretch gently, stopping before you feel discomfort. Repeat from the beginning. Move out of your final position, breathing calmly. Center your attention on your midsection, and take a final slow, deep breath. Repeat quietly to yourself: all is well... all is well... all is well.

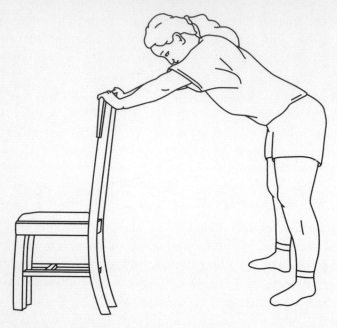

Begin standing, with your hands supported on a stable piece of furniture. Place your feet about shoulder-width apart and keep your head aligned with your spine.

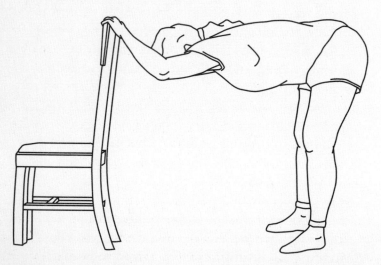

Slowly lower yourself from the waist, keeping your back straight, until you feel a gentle stretch along the back of the legs. Keep your head level with your back.

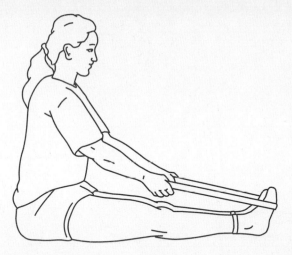

Begin seated, with your legs out in front of you. Place a flexible item over the bottom of your feet (such as a belt or towel), and hold the ends in your hands.

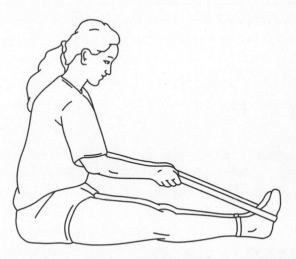

Sit up tall, lifting your ribs toward the ceiling. Gently bend forward from your waist until you feel a gentle stretch along the back of your legs. Be sure to avoid hunching your back or jutting your chin out in front of you. After holding the stretch for 20 to 30 seconds, slowly lower your chin to your chest until you feel a stretch along your back.

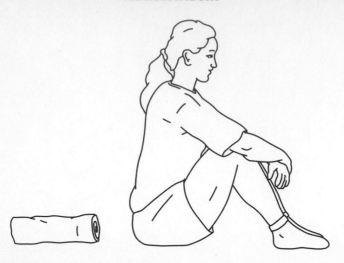

Place a rolled bath towel behind you so that when you lie down it will lie along your spine.

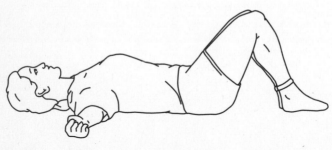

Slowly lie back over the towel so that the top of the towel is just below your shoulder blades. You should feel a gentle stretch in your chest muscles. You may lie in this position for as long as you wish, ideally for at least five minutes. If you are uncomfortable, you can change the intensity of the stretch by simply adjusting the size of the towel you use. When you are finished with this stretch, simply roll off the towel onto your side and carefully help yourself up.

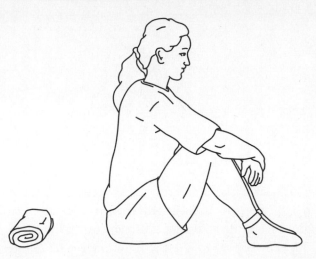

Turn the towel so that it will be perpendicular to your spine when you lie on it.

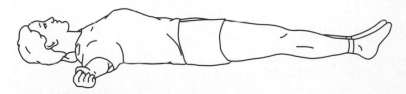

Lie back over the towel so that you feel a gentle stretch in your abdominal muscles. The towel should be just below your shoulder blades. You may lie in this position as long as you wish, and when you are ready to change positions, simply roll off the towel as you did in the previous stretch.

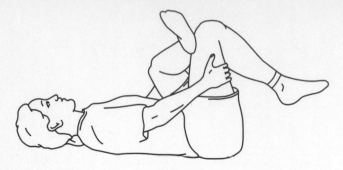

Lie on your back with knees bent. Cross your left ankle over your right knee. Place your hands behind each knee and gently pull your right knee toward your chest until you feel a gentle stretch in your hip. Lower your foot to the floor and repeat the stretch for the other side.

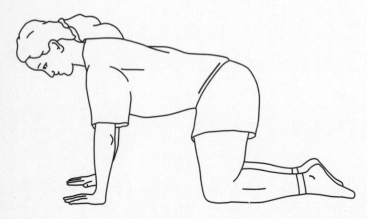

Begin on your hands and knees. (If you have knee pain, you may use a cushion under them.) Keep your head in line with your spine and allow your chest and stomach to settle toward the floor.

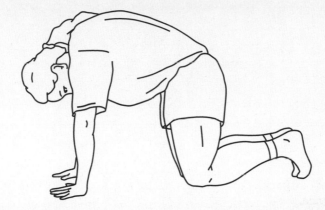

Imagine a string connected to your upper back that is pulling you up. Allow your head to relax downward while your hips press forward. Return to the starting position.

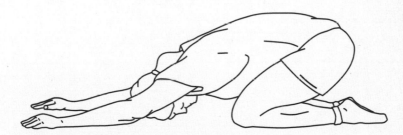

While on your hands and knees, push your hips back to your ankles, while keeping your hands in place. Allow your upper back and shoulders to lengthen and relax.

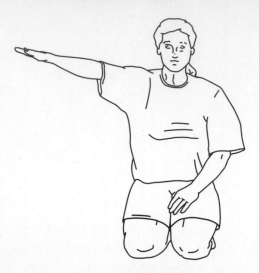

Come up to your knees. If you have problems with your knees, place a towel in the crease of your legs for support or do this stretch standing. Put one arm out to the side while relaxing your neck.

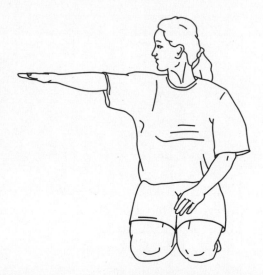

While either kneeling or standing, slowly turn your head toward the extended arm until you feel a gentle stretch in your neck. Keep your chin in a neutral position and avoid jutting it out over your shoulder. Return your head to the starting position and lower your arm. Repeat the stretch on the other side.

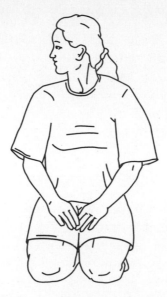

While either kneeling or standing, slowly turn your head to the right while keeping your chin in a neutral position.

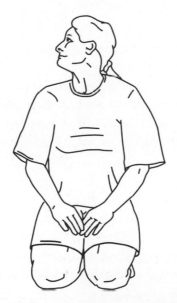

Gently extend your left jaw toward the ceiling until you feel a stretch along your chest, jaw, and temple. Repeat on the other side.

Once you get used to this style of stretching, you can use any position in which you feel tightness as a stretch. There's an old joke about a patient going to a doctor and saying, "Doctor, it hurts when I do this…" and the doctor replying, "Then don't do that." The doctor's new punch line (although significantly less funny) should be, "Well, then hold it there for 20 seconds while you breathe normally."

More Ways to Stretch

There are many other ways to get help with stretching, and over time you may want to incorporate a variety of them into your routine. There are excellent stretching classes available through local fitness centers and community education programs. It takes just one phone call to get a catalog, brochure, or other information to get you started.

You may also want to consider a videotape. By calling Collage Video at 1-800-433-6769, you can get their catalog of fitness videotapes, and they have a good selection to lead you through gentle stretching.

Other options include yoga and tai chi. Look for beginner classes or tapes and be sure they focus on flexibility or relaxation (as opposed to strength or endurance). If you are taking a class (as opposed to using a videotape), be sure to tell the instructor you have fibromyalgia. If they are not familiar with the condition, try to bring them some literature so they can familiarize themselves with how fibromyalgia might interact with the practice they are teaching you.

Diane is 37 and recently learned that her years of pain are due to fibromyalgia. Diane's doctor told her the only exercise she could do was in a warm-water pool. Her town had only one therapeutic pool, which was a 20-minute car ride from both her home and work place, but she was willing to try anything if it meant less pain.

She decided to make her first trip to the pool on the weekend. Her husband had agreed to watch their two children for the day, so she packed a bag with her bathing suit, towel, toiletries, and a change of clothes and set off to find the pool.

After 20 minutes in the pool, she thought she'd found heaven. Her pain began to ease, and she realized how much she missed being in the water. She lingered after swimming, taking her time in the shower and getting dressed. The rest of the day she felt like she was still floating in the water, and her pain noticeably improved.

After a couple of attempts to get to the pool on weekdays, Diane was getting frustrated. The pool wasn't open before she went to work. She made it there one afternoon after work, but because of her husband's work schedule she needed to be home by 5 P.M. to watch the kids and make dinner for the family. She felt rushed at the pool, and found that trying to get her bag together in the morning was an extra source of stress that made the whole thing seem like too much aggravation. "I can't live my whole life at the pool!" she thought. It seemed like her only choices were to be in constant pain or live out of a gym bag.

Diane knew there had to be another way. After doing some more reading, she realized that a heated pool wasn't the only way she could exercise. She learned that a heated pool is helpful because it provides nonimpact and gentle exercise but that other types of exercise also easily meet these criteria.

After rethinking her choices for movement, she decided the pool felt too good to give it up completely. Realistically, she could get to the pool one day over the weekend without feeling rushed or resentful.

On the weekdays, she received just as many benefits from a combination of walking, stretching, and using a tai chi videotape twice a week. She has significantly less pain than *she did before she got regular movement, and it's fitting easily into her life.*

In Review

Flexibility is just as important as activity and aerobic exercise for overall health and pain control.

Be sure to stretch your whole body five to seven times a week, and tight areas during the day as needed.

Be sure to use proper form when you stretch.

There are many ways to stretch. Don't be afraid to try something new!

CHAPTER 5

Fit Bodies Have Less Pain

Aerobic exercise: these two words are often the source of more misunderstanding and confusion than any other words related to exercise. There's even more confusion when people with fibromyalgia try to use exercise to help their condition. This chapter will help you understand the proper way to use aerobic exercise to help you manage the pain.

Before you even consider exercising, it's important that you are getting enough activity and sleeping well (see previous chapters). If you are not meeting your own activity needs and still try to exercise, you will have increased pain. Remember, exercise works through the breakdown of tissue combined with the ability of your body to rebuild itself stronger than it was before. And what happens when your body breaks down tissue and then sits very still? With fibromyalgia, your body responds by getting very stiff and very sore. And when you're stiff and sore, how likely are you to do more exercise? Take as much time as you need to increase your activity level. Just don't set yourself up for failure by trying to exercise too soon.

Now that I've talked you out of exercising and probably horrified your physician, let me make the case for getting aerobic exercise. Aerobic exercise is the closest thing to a medical magic bullet that's ever been found. Think you've heard all this before? Great! Here's your chance to show your stuff.

On a blank sheet of paper, write down as many benefits of getting aerobic exercise as you can. After you've written down every benefit you can think of, compare it with the list on the following pages.

Benefits of Aerobic Exercise

Increases endurance
Decreases fatigue
Improves sleep quality
Reduces risk of developing several types of cancer
Reduces risk of heart disease
Reduces risk of stroke
Increases longevity
Speeds recovery from illness
Strengthens immune system
Improves circulation
Improves arthritis
Improves fibromyalgia
Speeds recovery from surgery
Increases ability to burn fat as fuel
Improves diabetes
Can reduce or eliminate need for a wide variety of
    medications
Improves depression
Prevents depression
Improves and prevents panic attacks and other anxiety
    disorders
Reduces stress
Helps prevent stress
Reduces blood pressure
Helps prevent high blood pressure
Increases bone density
Helps prevent osteoporosis
Reduces cholesterol
Helps prevent elevated cholesterol
Improves multiple sclerosis
May slow progression of multiple sclerosis
Helps reverse heart disease
Helps prevent fat storage
Helps with weight loss

Reduces need for insulin and other medications used
   to treat diabetes
Improves success rates when quitting smoking
Reduces seasonal affective disorder
Eases stress of childbirth
Improves self-esteem
Improves body image
Increases body awareness
Improves self-confidence
Increases effectiveness of many other types of
   care
Helps improve headaches
Reduces PMS
Reduces menstrual cramps
Reduces menopause symptoms
Helps prevent delayed onset of diabetes
Improves irritable bowel disease
Improves diverticulitis
Improves seasonal allergies
Improves asthma
Reduces or eliminates need for asthma medications
Improves certain health aspects of chronic obstructive
   pulmonary disease
Reduces need for antidepressants
Reduces need for antianxiety medications
Decreases sugar cravings
Improves sense of well-being
Reduces need for caffeine
Improves sexual function and performance
Decreases resting heart rate
Decreases resting respiratory rate
Enables heart to pump more blood with each stroke
Increases amount of oxygen carried in the blood
Enhances creativity in all areas
Reduces number of sick days
Improves memory

How'd you do? How did you feel when you compared your list with the one on the preceding pages? Were you surprised? Most people have a vague sense that exercise is good for them but have no idea of the number of benefits there is to receive from it.

Now go back and star the items in the list that are especially important to you as a person with fibromyalgia. Be careful here. Don't limit your thinking to the obvious connection to your muscles and pain level. Be sure to think about the other implications. You may not think preventing osteoporosis is related to fibromyalgia, but what happens if you break a hip and have to lie around for eight weeks recovering from hip-replacement surgery? How many items seem to apply to you? Do you still think aerobic exercise is only for losing weight?

Although aerobic exercise can dramatically reduce the pain of fibromyalgia, you have to do it right, and doing it right means making sure you follow certain guidelines. A more detailed explanation is provided later in the chapter, but following are the key points you should keep in mind while exercising. Some of these are different for people without fibromyalgia and some aren't. Keep these concepts in mind at all times, especially when you are beginning or making changes to your exercise program, because these are the times you will be most vulnerable to flare-ups.

Key Points to Remember about Aerobic Exercise

- Avoid impact. Impact is any motion that has you jumping and landing with a force harder than normal walking. Doing exercise that includes moderate-to high-impact movements is almost never well tolerated by people with fibromyalgia. Examples of high-impact exercise are jogging, aerobic dance (not specifically designated as low impact), double-footed jump roping, jumping jacks, and similar movements.

This type of movement almost always causes muscles affected with fibromyalgia to spasm and harden. If this happens, refer to Chapter 10 on managing flare-ups and then try to avoid that type of movement again.

- Vary your movements and positions. Some exercises such as riding a bike require you to stay in a fixed position for an extended period of time, and this can aggravate your pain. You may find it helpful to spend short amounts of time on a few different activities. If you are exercising at a gym, this may mean spending 10 minutes on the bike, 10 minutes on the treadmill, and another 10 on a stair-climbing machine. If you exercise at home, this may mean combining your bike riding with a walk. Again, listen to your body. If the first few minutes on a bike are fine and then you feel pain in your neck, back, or hip, stop and switch to something else. If you can stay on a bike for an extended period of time with no ill effects, then there's no need to change activities every 10 minutes.

- Avoid movements that rely on the areas most affected by your fibromyalgia. Do you have lots of neck and shoulder pain from fibromyalgia? Then you might want to skip the rowing machine and water skiing. You may also find that lap swimming and aerobic dance are too strenuous on your neck. Walking is a great place to start, but be sure to use proper form (more on this later).

- To get the benefits of aerobic exercise, make sure your exercise is aerobic. This means that the movement you choose increases your heart rate to a comfortable but elevated level for at least 15 minutes. The more intense an exercise is, the less amount of time you need to do it to get aerobic benefits. Since this book focuses on pain management for fibromyalgia, I'm going to encourage you to choose low-intensity, long-duration exercise. This is less likely to cause a flare-up and will give you the most pain relief. As you get fit, you may want to experiment with more intense exercise. If you are just beginning, start gently.

- Never start or stop exercising abruptly. This means don't go from being sedentary to jumping into a full exercise program without working up to it gradually. Also, don't stop a regular exercise program suddenly and become sedentary. Unless, of course, you don't mind debilitating pain.

How Hard Should You Exercise?

When people ask how hard they should exercise, they're really asking about one of the variables of exercise: *intensity*. There are a lot of charts available that show a range for your heart rate to stay within, and if you find these helpful and easy to use, please do so. However, there is a fair amount of variance from person to person with target heart rates, and most of us don't have this chart with us when we exercise anyway.

There's a simpler and more accurate way to gauge how hard you are exercising. Think of it as a 1 to 10 scale with 10 being running for your life (as hard as possible) and 1 being the pace at which you might browse through a store. At 2, 3, or 4, you are able to speak easily and in complete sentences. You could also sing at this level. At 5, 6, and 7 you can talk, but after every few words you take a breath or two. You could not sing at this level of intensity, but can maintain this level comfortably. By the time you reach 8, 9, or 10, you start to gasp for breath and can't maintain this level for very long. When you are exercising, you want to be at a level of 5, 6, or 7 on this scale. Your warm-up and cool-down should be in the range of 2 to 3 and can simply be a slower version of the movement you're doing for exercise, for 3 to 5 minutes. You can change activities for the warm-up and cool-down, but it is not necessary.

Intensity Scale

1. Very gentle movement, such as browsing in a store.
2. Steady, but leisurely.
3. Steady but comfortable work, such as taking an evening stroll.
4. Quick pace, but not out of breath.
5. More intense, such as a brisk walk. May need to interrupt conversation with extra breaths.
6. Moderately intense. Conversation is interrupted every few words with extra breaths.
7. Increasingly intense, but still comfortable.
8. Getting very intense. Cannot hold a conversation or maintain intensity for very long.
9. Miserably strenuous.
10. The absolute maximum your body can do, such as running from something dangerous.

The second variable with aerobic exercise is *duration.* I stress again the importance of having a strong foundation of activity before you begin exercising. The guideline I'm recommending is based on the assumption that you have that crucial part of managing your fibromyalgia in place. If you are getting at least 60 minutes of activity in your day with decent pain control and your doctor has cleared you to exercise, you can safely begin with 15 minutes of exercise including the warm-up and cool-down.

As this level of duration becomes more comfortable, you can increase it in increments of 5 minutes. Is there an upper limit for duration? Yes and no. For pain management, you'll be getting about all the benefits you can from aerobic movement in about 40 to 60 minutes. However, this is the real world, so you may hit your upper limit at 30 minutes because of pain, time limits, or some other issue. The minimum is more important for pain control than the maximum. Shoot for a minimum of 15 to 20 minutes. This will allow the systemic changes that come with aerobic exercise to start happening. Because you will most likely be doing low-intensity aerobic exercise, you'll need to do it longer to get the aerobic benefits. If you'd like more in-depth information about this, Covert Bailey has written the best books I've ever seen on the topic, and they are listed in the recommended reading list at the end of this book.

The last variable is *frequency*. This has to do with how often you exercise. The standard three to four times a week will be good enough for many people with fibromyalgia, but it's not uncommon for people to need more than this. You may get your best pain relief on the days you exercise, and assuming you don't have a reason not to, you can exercise seven days a week.

Now before you throw the book across the room and sign me off as someone totally out of touch with the real world, let me explain what I mean by exercising seven days a week. I'm not talking about running 10 miles a day, seven days a week. I'm not talking about taking an aerobic dance class seven days a week or having to go to a gym to exercise. Remember that the exercise we're talking about is gentle, easy, and comfortable. It could even be done twice a day if desired. If it's a busy day, walking out your front door and coming back 15 to 20 minutes later might be your exercise for the day. Assuming you have the time for it, there's no problem with doing this every day once you've worked up to it. Go gradually and listen to your body. It won't take long for you to know which frequency works best for you.

The Importance of Form

What do exercise experts mean when they talk about using proper form? When referring to aerobic exercise, using good form means exercising in a way that helps you do the movement effectively without aggravating another part of your body.

Let's look at walking as a simple example. When you walk, what is your form like? In other words, how are you positioning your body when you walk? Where is your chin? Tucked in toward your chest or jutted out ahead of your body? How about your hips? Tucked under or pointed out? Are you swinging your arms? How long is your stride? All of these considerations are especially important for people with fibromyalgia. If your form is poor, it can cause new pain in joints and muscles that will throw off your exercise program.

Here are some general tips for keeping good form while exercising:

- Keep your chin tucked in toward your chest to avoid straining your neck.
- Keep your abdominal muscles firm to support your torso, but not so tight that your breathing is restricted.
- Center yourself in your body and avoid leaning forward or backward while in motion.
- Be sure to breathe from your abdomen and not your chest.

How Do I Know What to Do for Exercise?

There are many types of aerobic exercise. The general guidelines given in this chapter can easily be applied to any type of aerobic exercise, and when combined with your knowledge about your body, should be able to keep you in line. And because variety in an exercise program is crucial to having fun, staying motivated, and not overworking certain parts of your body, you will often need to think about form. Here are some more specific tips on common aerobic exercises and good form. If something you do is not listed here, you can follow the general guidelines in this chapter. Play with it on your own, or consider consulting an exercise specialist for personalized help.

Walking
Walking is one of the best forms of exercise for a variety of reasons: it's cheap, easy to do, and can be done by almost anyone. But despite how easy it is, when done incorrectly, walking can be

painful. Done correctly, however, walking can ease the pain of fibromyalgia with little risk of causing a flare-up. You may want to walk while someone reads this to you, so you can concentrate on your body and make adjustments as the suggestions are being read to you.

First, start off slowly and gradually pick up the pace over the first several minutes. Starting too quickly can strain muscles, ligaments, or tendons, which once injured can take a long time to heal. Remember the 1 to 10 scale? Starting slowly means being at level 1 or 2 and gradually working up from there over five to seven minutes. The following are some other things to keep in mind.

- Try to avoid overswinging your arms. This can aggravate muscles in the neck and cause pain.
- Keep your elbows close to your body and bend them to about a 90-degree angle. This helps take the pressure off your neck.
- As your pace increases, take shorter, quicker steps. Taking longer steps is a primary cause of pain in the shin and throws off your form considerably. Shorter steps also allow you to go faster with less impact on your body

Swimming

Many people with fibromyalgia get at least some of their exercise in a pool. It's so popular for fibromyalgia patients that some doctors have begun to think it's the only exercise they can do. Not true! It is true that warm-water pools offer a nonimpact, relaxing workout, but you are in no way limited to this option. In fact, if you do limit yourself to just swimming, you are going to be so fed up with the whole ritual of packing your pool bag, driving to the pool, changing, swimming, showering, drying off, getting dressed, driving home, and unpacking your wet things that after two weeks you may be likely to, shall we say, throw in the towel. Keep it simple because you're going to be exercising most days of the week. Swimming can be a part of your routine, but not the only part.

Using good form while swimming depends on what you are doing once you're in the water. If you are swimming laps, it's crucial that your upper body is strong enough to handle this without spasming into knots. If you are new to swimming, especially if you are not on medications to help your restorative sleep, I don't recommend lap swimming.

If, however, you are doing what a friend of mine calls bobbing around in the water, you can keep good form more easily. The best way to make this an aerobic workout is to wear pool footwear, which is essentially slippers with tub grips to give you traction on the pool bottom, and walk through chest-deep water. Keep your arms underwater and move them as you would when walking on dry land. Bringing them up above the water level can stress your neck, which defeats the point of exercising to reduce pain. Keep your shoulders relaxed and have the movement originate from your legs.

Another option is to take a water-aerobic class, which can be great for new exercisers who aren't quite sure what they should be doing out there. The advantage of this type of aerobics class is that it's totally nonimpact, and you have an instructor watching your form for you. And there's a good chance you'll meet other people trying to manage chronic pain, just like you.

Aerobic Dance

In order to get and keep your heart rate elevated, aerobic dance classes rely heavily on lots of arm movements and varied body positions. As you get more fit, these movements tend to get more intense to keep you in your aerobic zone, and they can often aggravate fibromyalgia pain to the point that you'd swear exercise is bad for you. The upside is that for most people aerobic dance is fun; it is done to music and is so varied it's hard to get bored. It has all the elements of a great exercise option. If you choose to include it as one of your exercise options, keep the following in mind.

- Beware of aggravating your neck. While you adjust to the movements, keep your wrists below your shoulders. This means you'll be modifying many of the arm motions shown to you. As you get stronger, you can experiment with slowly adding in movements that take your wrists above your shoulders. Unless you are willing to deal with flare-ups as you learn what you can and can't do with aerobic dance, go very slowly. If you are taking a class with an instructor (versus a videotaped class) talk with the instructor about your fibromyalgia and ask for suggestions on modifying the moves and if he or she can work with you during class. You may even be able to find, or suggest your exercise facility create, a class just for people with fibromyalgia.
- Keep your knees over your ankles. When bending your knees, never let them extend over or beyond your feet. This greatly overstresses the knees and back and can cause all kinds of problems. Keeping your weight on the front of your heel (versus the back of your heel or ball of your foot) will also help you stay in line when bending at the knees.
- Remember to breathe and stay relaxed while you dance.
- Many aerobic dance classes have a section of floor work, which is actually muscle conditioning. Unless you are really ready to begin this type of exercise, don't do this part of the class. Use the time to stretch.

Aerobic dance on videotape can be an excellent way to make exercise more convenient. It also offers more privacy than a gym and is relatively inexpensive. Even people with the smallest of spaces in front of their TVs can make use of most tapes. I've had great luck using exercise videotapes, and having a variety of them on hand keeps my interest up. I can pick the tape according to my energy and pain level of the day. The trick is finding good ones. There are lots of effective, safe tapes available, but they can be harder to find than the glitzy celebrity ones. This is not to say that if a tape has a celebrity in it that it's not a good tape, but that most of the really great ones don't have any celebrities.

Collage Video, based in Minneapolis, has a mail-order service that is outstanding. Their phones are staffed with exercise professionals who have tried the tapes and can match your needs to one or more of their tapes. For a free catalog, call 1-800-433-6769.

Biking/Bike Machines

Whether you are using a traditional bike or a stationary one, the main issue with form is being sure the bike fits you and the seat and handlebars are adjusted correctly. If you are buying the bike new, be sure to talk to the salesperson for help with this. If you already have a bike, you need to double-check the seat height. The general rule is that when sitting on the seat with one leg all the way down, your leg is extended, but there's still a slight bend in the knee. The same guidelines work for recumbent bikes, where your legs are out in front of you rather than underneath and which are much easier on the neck and lower back.

Cross-Country Skiing/Ski Machines

This exercise option is great for people with fibromyalgia because it is so gentle and works virtually every muscle in the body at once. The machines do a great job of imitating the real thing, but nothing compares to how it feels to be gliding through the snow in the winter woods.

Regardless of where you ski, indoors or out, good form means taking moderate-size strides, maintaining a comfortable pace, and keeping your balance in the center of your body. In colder climates during winter, many parks and recreation areas offer cross-country skiing lessons where you can get instruction on proper form. Cross-country skiing is very similar to walking, and you can get good enough to use it for mild exercise with minimal instruction.

Shoes

Sometimes one solution to the pain problem can be found by simply looking down at your shoes. There's no question that in any field there are a lot of people trying to sell you equipment you don't need at very high prices. Exercise is no exception, but shoes are one item in which you will need to invest some money or pay the higher price of increased pain and injury. I've worked with patients who experienced various types of pain. I wish I could count all the times I asked them what kind of condition their shoes were in and they said, "Oh, they still look fine. They're only two years old." However, how athletic shoes look has nothing to do with what kind of condition they are in, but rather how much they've been used. And to a certain point, you do get what you pay for with athletic shoes.

Shoes made for performance and not just looks have some very specific features, such as cushioning devices, arch supports, cooling vents, and padding, which don't last forever. The shoes can look fine, but if you've used them regularly for 6 to 12 months, it's probably time for new ones. Athletic shoes are designed to last a certain number of hours; after that, they simply don't perform as they used to. When you buy athletic shoes, ask the salesperson what the life expectancy is if they are used a certain number of times a week, and this will give you a ballpark figure for when you need to replace them. Once the shoes are retired from exercise, you don't necessarily need to toss them out. They may still be great for running errands, as a spare pair, or for gardening, but they should be retired from regular exercise.

Another key point often missed is that there really are differences between shoes for running and walking, aerobic dance, tennis, and any other type of exercise. Every activity has certain moves that are common to it. Walking puts a great deal of pressure down on the heel and then into a forward roll, but uses very little side-to-side motion. Aerobic dance, by contrast, is almost all side-to-side motion and very little movement that resembles walking. To accommodate this, each shoe is made for a certain sport or activity and should not be used for one it wasn't made for.

So, what's this going to cost you? A good shoe, regardless of what type of exercise it is for, will range from $50 to $100. Pay any more than that and you may be spending more than you need to;

pay any less and you might not be getting the quality you need. Be on the lookout for sales. Be willing to try on several pairs and call around for the best price. If you walk and do aerobic dance and pool walking, see if you can receive a discount for buying three pairs at once. Stick with name brands, be sure you're buying shoes made for your gender, and have a salesperson help you get a good fit. They'll inevitably suggest their most expensive shoe first, so feel free to give them a price range you are comfortable with. Here are some general tips:

- Know your price range.
- Try on several different brands of shoes for the particular exercise you plan to do.
- Always try on shoes after you've been up and around for several hours. Feet swell throughout the day, and if you buy shoes first thing in the morning you're likely to buy shoes that won't fit later.
- Talk to the salesperson about the type of exercise you plan to do, along with any other particulars about your feet, such as if you tend to walk on one side of your foot, have medical problems with your feet, or have wide or narrow feet or high or low arches.
- Ask how long you can expect the shoe to last.
- Wear the socks you will be exercising in when you try on shoes.
- Be sure your feet have room in the shoe. They should feel comfortable from the moment you put them on. Athletic shoes should not have to be broken in.
- If the salesperson can't answer your questions, go somewhere else.
- Take your time in the store. Walk around, jump, and do anything else that simulates the exercise you'll be doing in the shoes.

Elizabeth is 65 and was told she had fibromyalgia 10 years ago. She had been sedentary most of her life and was overweight. When she attempted to lose weight, she cut her caloric intake to less than 1,200 per day and did not exercise. Chronic pain had been a way of life literally for decades.

When she decided to try increasing her movement, she started with stretching. She noticed she felt better immediately after she stretched, but the effect lasted only an hour or two. She was willing to cut down on her time spent motionless, but she didn't know what to do with herself once she stood up. She was retired, widowed, and had no family that lived near her.

She called the senior center in her community and learned that they offered senior exercise classes. She began with water aerobics twice a week. She noticed she had her best days when she went to the pool for a couple of hours in the morning. She also noticed she slept best on those nights.

After a month of stretching and swimming, she and another woman from her class decided to walk together on their days off from the pool. Elizabeth was younger than her new walking partner, and they both were concerned that they would have different paces when they walked. Elizabeth suggested that she walk over to the house of her classmate because it was a couple blocks away and that they go together from there. When they were done Elizabeth would walk home. This allowed Elizabeth to have a longer walk where she could set the pace, but to still spend time with her friend and have the support of exercising with someone.

Elizabeth still has bad days and occasional flare-ups, but she rarely feels incapacitated by the fibromyalgia. She can't imagine spending long days reading and watching TV, paralyzed with pain. She has lost 15 pounds since she started exercising six months ago, and she is hopeful that she will continue to slowly lose excess fat as she gets stronger and more active.

Maria has never been able to imagine life without exercise. She's an aerobics instructor and competitive runner and has been active in sports since high school. She finds it increasing-

ly difficult to train due to dramatic increases in her fibro-myalgia pain. She is constantly tired and knows she isn't sleep-ing well. She wants to avoid taking medications for her sleep, but doesn't know what else to do. After speaking to an herbal-ist, she decided to try an herb to help her sleep at night. After three weeks, she noticed she was sleeping better, but the pain had not improved. Her doctor recommended she cut her exer-cise in half for a couple weeks to see if pain improved. Although it meant not teaching any aerobics classes and drop-ping out of her next race, she was willing to try.

The difference was immediate. The combination of more rest, less strenuous exercise, and better sleep allowed Maria's body to heal at night and not constantly aggravate the fibro-myalgia during her workouts.

Now she had a tough decision. It was clear her body did better with more moderate movement, but she didn't want to give up teaching aerobics and running races. She thought about her health and her choices and decided that she would still race, but cut her race schedule to two races a year instead of five. She still wanted to teach fitness classes, so she offered to teach a stretching class and limited her aerobics instruc-tion to one class per week.

With her extra time, she started exploring other ways to ease her pain without compromising her fitness level. She started taking yoga, which she loved from the first class, added in muscle conditioning twice a week, and hiked on hilly trails near her home. She also found a good massage therapist whom she sees twice a month to help release her neck and shoulders, especially around race time. Her pain has improved to the point that it hardly ever bothers her, and things seem less of a struggle now. She is willing to deal with extra pain after a race as a compromise with her body and the fibromyalgia.

There's no question that aerobic exercise, if done correctly, can improve nearly every aspect of your life. Don't miss one of the most powerful ways you have to heal your mind, body, and spirit by spending all your energy on finding reasons not to exercise.

In Review

Be sure you are satisfying your activity needs before you begin exercising.

Start gradually and never start or stop an exercise program abruptly.

Aerobic exercise can drastically improve many aspects of your health and your pain.

Follow the general exercise guidelines in this chapter and apply them to any type of aerobic exercise you do.

Follow the guidelines in this chapter for intensity, duration, and frequency of exercise for best pain relief. Exercise should be comfortable enough that you can work up to exercising every day.

Use proper form when you exercise.

Have a variety of aerobic exercises to choose from to keep things interesting for you and your body. There are lots of resources and opportunities to explore out there.

Make sure you have shoes that are designed specifically for what you plan to do, are in good condition internally, and fit you well.

CHAPTER 6

Strong Bodies
Have Less Pain

Let's do a little experiment. I'm going to present a word (actually it's two words) to you, and I'd like you to clear your mind and see what image you get when you read it. Ready? *Weight lifting*. What image did you see? For most people, the image that comes to mind is a sweaty male who is so enormous he can't even turn his head.

Let's try the experiment again, this time with a few more words. Picture a woman. She has a healthy body weight for her height and build and is lean and toned. When she waves hello to you, her upper arm doesn't wave back. When she lifts a child, it's clear she feels strong and solid. In the spring, she gardens and can lift large bags of soil with little effort. There's a strong flex in her arms and legs when she moves, and she rarely feels stiff and sore. She always seems to be able to eat heartily without gaining excess body fat. This is a weight lifter.

Weight lifting is one of the best-kept secrets in women's health. For too long, men have been the only ones getting the countless benefits of muscle conditioning, while women have been packed in the aerobics room getting frustrated with their progress. Muscle conditioning is finally starting to get the long-overdue attention from women.

In case you are wondering what all the fuss is about, you're not alone. Why bother doing it? That's a good question. Let's start by clearing up the main fear I hear from women when the topic of muscle conditioning comes up. You will not, I repeat, will *not* bulk up, look like a man, and have veins popping out of your neck. With the exception of a very few individuals and those foolish enough to use steroids, women simply do not have the physical makeup to get so muscular that they pop out of their clothes. And if you are one of those rare women who gains muscle mass easily, lucky you! Muscle conditioning is one of the main ways to increase your fitness quickly. Fit bodies have less pain.

Muscle conditioning also helps the pain of fibromyalgia in other ways. Strong muscles better support painful joints. Well-conditioned muscles make it much easier to have good posture and keep your body in proper alignment. You won't get as tired with a strong set of muscles.

Muscle conditioning gets very specific muscles moving and keeps much-needed blood and oxygen flowing freely to your muscles, nourishing them fully. Strong muscles have more endurance and resist spasm more readily.

There are still more ways muscle conditioning helps fibromyalgia. Out of your entire body, your muscles consume the most calories. It is similar to sitting down to a family dinner and having your giant cousin Lou hoard all the food before anyone else can get any. Your muscles are like your cousin Lou. They use a ton of calories while your fat sits quietly at the end of the table and nibbles on lettuce. If you have a lot of muscle on your body, you burn dramatically more calories during the day. This means you lose weight and become resistant to gaining excess body fat. Did you hear that? *Resistant* to gaining body fat!

How about some numbers to help convince you? Every pound of extra muscle you add to your body takes another 30 to 50 calories per day just to maintain it. If you were to add just 5 pounds of muscle to your body (which can be done in a couple of months), you burn an *extra* 3,000 to 7,000 calories a month, which is equal to 1 to 2 pounds of body fat lost in that month. And that's without changing anything else! And it's no secret how helpful it is to lose excess body fat when you have fibromyalgia.

Starting at age 30, we lose 2 percent of our muscle mass *every year* unless we are doing muscle conditioning to maintain it. This means that every year you gain weight more easily even though you eat about the same. Every year you have more and more pain because your precious muscle is wasting away while you find reasons not to exercise. Over the years, I have worked with many patients in exactly this position who still cling to the old, worn-out excuses like, "I don't have time," "I'll do it later," and "Someday I'll get to it." Don't let this be you! If you are over 30, this muscle loss is happening to you right now. If you are well over 30, it's been happening for years, and you need to stop it now and start reversing the clock on your muscles and your pain. And if you're under 30 and figure you have a couple years to go before you have to worry about all this, why wait until there's a problem? You can get a head start and hit age 30 with *extra* muscle, and you'll hardly notice the effects of this age-related muscle wasting.

I feel obligated to tell you that there are experts who recommend that people with fibromyalgia do not lift weights. Ever. They have accurately observed that after lifting weights, people with fibromyalgia often experience an immediate and dramatic increase in pain.

It is my opinion that this is often due to poor sleep quality (which is when your body does the bulk of the repair work after lifting weights) and lifting incorrectly. I have seen many people get stronger, leaner, and reduce the pain of fibromyalgia with muscle conditioning *if* they are getting healthy sleep *and* are lifting the weights exactly as I have described. I strongly encourage you to add muscle conditioning to your fibromyalgia care plan at the appropriate time and in the proper way.

Now before you drop to the ground and start cranking out sit-ups and push-ups, let's talk about the basics. When you lift a weight several times, you break down the muscle being worked. When you're done exhausting your muscle, it starts to repair itself. It's as though it says, "I'm going to repair the tissue a little bit stronger than it was before so I can handle it if she does that again." If you don't use the muscle in a similar way relatively soon, your body assumes it was a one-time freak occurrence and doesn't bother to maintain the gain. But, if you work the muscle two to three times a week, your body will continually adapt and get stronger, and you'll get all the benefits of muscle conditioning. Unless you're not sleeping well…

You knew there had to be a catch, didn't you? Much of the adapting and tissue repair happens, you guessed it, during the exact stage of sleep that people with fibromyalgia tend to miss. So, what will happen if you start strength conditioning when restorative sleep is still not in place? You'll have more than just normal soreness 24 to 48 hours after exercise. Muscle conditioning without proper sleep can potentially trigger pain flares that can be difficult to control.

If you are not getting restorative sleep you should not be doing strength conditioning. Period. As I mentioned earlier in the book, if you are not getting quality sleep, that should be your first priority over any formal exercise plan. However, once your doctor has given you permission to exercise, you shouldn't have any problems if your sleep is normal and you lift with care. Remember that you are lifting for health, not so you can compete in the Olympics. Go easy.

Many people believe that the only way to do strength conditioning is to join a gym and spend hours working each muscle. Not only is this not true, but I want to adamantly forbid you from doing this. We've learned a lot about muscle conditioning since the old days, and you'll have no problem doing your muscle conditioning at home if you choose to do so.

I have deliberately not included specific muscle conditioning exercises here for a couple of reasons. First, I've never had good luck with just using pictures and brief descriptions to teach someone how to lift weights. Form is crucial to getting results and not causing a pain flare, and I'm not convinced pictures can give you what you need.

Second, if you have any other injuries or weak areas on your body (such as lower back pain or bad knees) there is a real risk of aggravating these problems. You need better coaching on options if the pictured exercise doesn't work for you.

Last, there are so many different ways to work each muscle, both in a gym and at home, that it would be more confusing than helpful to try and list all the options here. I will provide you with ideas and resources so that you can decide what will work best.

Using a Gym

Many people choose to do strength conditioning at a gym. The main advantages of doing it at a gym are (1) every piece of equipment you need is in one place, and (2) you have access to weight-lifting machines and trainers. The downsides are that it costs money to join a gym and you have to go there to use it, which tends to chew up a fair amount of time. The most common way to do muscle conditioning at a gym is to use free weights or machines made specifically for muscle conditioning.

Maybe you're not a member of a gym but have been considering joining one. I'm often asked what to look for when joining a gym, and there are certainly several key things to check out. One thing is for sure, if you have not given clear thought to how this membership will fit into your life, you won't use it. Don't purchase a gym membership on impulse or get talked into a special price that's going to expire in the next 24 hours. Some other things to consider include the following:

Price. Know your price range before you go in to check things out. Call a few gyms you are considering and get price quotes. Visit the two or three that are in your range, and don't set foot in the others. There are some very nice gyms available, and they often have prices that are just as eye-popping. If you can reasonably afford it, it may be the perfect facility for you. Just don't fall into the "If it's really expensive, I'll be more motivated to use it" trap. Much of the time, the prices and the sign-up fees for gym memberships are negotiable. Extra months can oftentimes be used as currency, so haggle until you are happy. Be sure to read the fine print and know the terms of the contract.

Location. If the gym isn't conveniently located to you, you won't use it. Don't try to convince yourself otherwise.

Facilities. If you know you plan to use weight-lifting machines or any other specific equipment, be sure the gym has it. Not all gyms have the same facilities. Don't let a muscular salesperson tell you they plan to add a pool next year so why not sign up. Make sure the gym has what you want when you join. Check out the locker room and equipment for cleanliness and upkeep. Ask about the gym's hours and class schedules and be sure they match what you want. Current gym members are often selling their memberships for much less than the regular price. Before you sign up through the gym, check out your local paper to see if someone is trying to sell his or her membership and negotiate your best price with him or her. It could save you a significant amount of money.

Visit the gym during the time you plan to go. Gyms definitely have slow and busy times. Can you get near the equipment you plan to use at the time you want to use it?

On-site trainers. If you think you might consider a personal trainer, see what the gym's stock looks like, along with the prices. Be sure the trainers are certified and are familiar with fibromyalgia. Most gyms won't let you bring your own trainer into their facility.

Sales pitch. Don't allow yourself to be pressured by the sales staff. A quality club will not corner you and will let you see or try the club without signing up. Tell them if you are feeling pressured. Ask if they'll give you a two-week pass so you can see if it's really going to work for you. Most places are happy to accommodate this request; if not, ask them why.

Child care. Many gyms offer child care, and if this is a service you'll be using, you'll want to check it out as you would any other baby-sitter. Who staffs their day care? What is the staff-per-child ratio? Is there a cost for the service? What are the hours?

Once you've got your new membership, you'll want to be sure you don't hurt yourself lifting weights on the first day and need three months to recover. If you are not familiar with the machines or weights, do not saunter into the weight room and start playing around with them. Sign up for a meeting with a staff member for an introduction, and let him or her show you how to use the machines correctly. A one-time consultation should not cost you anything, and there should be no obligation on your part to purchase additional training sessions. Be sure the person you meet with is certified to teach muscle conditioning and that you feel comfortable with him or her.

The trainer should spend at least half an hour with you and get a thorough health and exercise history from you. Then you should be trained on each exercise you plan to do.

Here's a checklist you can take to be sure you get all your questions answered:

Weightlifting Checklist

- I have been given 10 to 14 exercises that target the major muscle groups in my body.
- I have been taught what resistance level to use for each exercise.
- I have been shown how to adjust machines to fit my body such as seat heights and pad angles.
- I have been told when to increase the weight.
- I have been shown correct form for each exercise, including range of motion, speed during all phases of the motion, and proper breathing.
- I know how many sets and reps to do.
- I know how each exercise should feel.
- I know where to go if I have questions.

I will provide some of this information for you in the following pages, but be sure to fill in any gaps with your trainer.

Getting Stronger at Home

If you decide gym life isn't for you, take heart! You can do a very effective muscle conditioning routine in your home, and it doesn't require a giant home gym machine. The only things you'll need are a few weights, and a videotape or a trainer.

You can buy weights at major retailers and sporting goods stores, and they aren't prohibitively expensive for most people. If you go this route, be sure to compare prices before you buy. There's no need to pay for extra features. You can start with a couple of 2-pound weights and progress from there. If you've been exercising for a while, 3 to 5 pounds might be a better starting place.

But even before you start shopping, consider other things that could be used as weights that might be sitting in your house right now. Do you have two large soup cans? They'll get you started. Two water bottles can work wonderfully as weights and be adjusted by simply filling or draining out some of the water. These options work just as well as purchased hand weights, especially when you are first getting started.

I mentioned that you'd also need a videotape because most people don't know what to do with the weights once they get them. And one of the key rules in exercise is: when lifting weights, form is everything. With aerobic exercise, as long as you're moving and keeping your heart rate where it should be, it doesn't matter how it looks. You can roll around, chase your dog, or have your limbs flying every which way and it won't affect the workout or the results. Not so with weight lifting. When you work to condition your muscles, it takes a certain amount of concentration, and you have to do it right or else you'll end up in pain and no stronger. If you can afford the luxury of a personal trainer, by all means do so! Many will come right to your home and show you how to do strength conditioning without joining a gym. But most of us will need to find another way to be sure our form is right, and that's why videotapes are perfect. For about $20, you can mirror perfect form and be guided through a variety of different movements. As you get more familiar with the movements, you can certainly do the exercises without the tape on, but until then don't try to figure it out on your own. Your time is valuable, so be sure you're investing it wisely.

Maybe you're thinking, "Sounds fine. But where do I find a videotape, and how can I be sure I'm getting a good one?" As I mentioned in the chapter about aerobic exercise, there's a wonderful resource for exercise videos that takes almost all the guesswork out of it. You can get a catalog from Collage Video by calling 1-800-433-6769. They have a whole section of videotapes just on muscle conditioning, and each tape is thoroughly described. You'll want a tape specifically for beginners that targets the whole body. There are several good ones available, and the staff at Collage will even help you pick one.

The Next Step

So now you have the tape and your weights, or have joined a gym or hired a trainer. Now what? This is one of those areas in which people with fibromyalgia need to do things a little bit differently than people without. The standard recommendations are to do muscle conditioning two to four times a week, each time working the muscle you are using to exhaustion. This means to lift the weight until you can't lift it one more time and still keep good form. The heavier the weight, the sooner this happens, and it's suggested that you reach muscle failure in 8 to 12 repetitions of the motion. Once you have reached this point, you have done one set. Although there's a fair amount of controversy right now about how many sets you need to do, most agree that one to three sets will get you there. But because you have fibromyalgia, these recommendations will need to be changed a little.

You should start with muscle conditioning two days a week, and only perform one set of each exercise. Aim to use a weight that allows you to lift it 12 to 14 times before your muscle starts to tire. Lastly, do not work to the point of muscle failure, at which you absolutely cannot lift the weight one more time and your muscles feel like wet noodles. Instead, you want to work your muscles to the point of fatigue. This is the point at which you can feel your muscles getting weaker, but you could do one or two more repetitions if you pushed.

When you are lifting the weight, focus your attention on the muscle being worked. Try to relax all other muscles in your body except the one(s) you are using.

Don't rush! Inhale. Exhale and lift the weight in two counts, hold for one count. Inhale and return to the starting position in four counts. When you are counting, you are not counting seconds (1-Mississippi, 2-Mississippi, and so on). You can simply count "1 and 2 and 3," and so on.

It should all come together like this:

- Get into position. Adjust the machine and your body for the movement and choose your resistance level.
- Relax your entire body.
- Inhale.
- Tense only the muscle you are about to use.
- Exhale and lift the weight in about two counts.
- Hold in top position briefly.
- Inhale and return to starting position in four counts.
- Without resting or releasing the muscle being worked, repeat until the exercised muscle is fatigued.
- When that muscle is fatigued, move on to the next exercise until you have worked all the major areas of your body.

Why You Need Special Care

Why do people with fibromyalgia need to lift weights differently than usually recommended? There are a few reasons, all of which have to do with reducing your pain. By lifting only two times a week, you give your muscles plenty of time to repair themselves before you work them again. By using lighter weights at higher repetitions, you reduce the risk for strain, injury, and pain flares, but still get results that make it worthwhile. Lastly, by working to the point of fatigue instead of failure, you avoid some of the face and neck straining that often comes with the last couple of repetitions.

If you follow these guidelines for two month's without any additional pain, you can increase the different variables one at a time and in this order: start by increasing the frequency to three times a week, and if that feels comfortable, begin to increase the weights and decrease the reps. If you're still hanging in there, then try working to exhaustion instead of just to fatigue. I don't recommend that fibromyalgia patients try to lift weights four days a week, no matter how well they're doing, simply because the risk of causing a flare is so great. If you decide to try it, don't increase the weights at the same time. Go slowly.

You often see people without fibromyalgia (at least I hope they don't have it) being coached to really push themselves when they lift weights. They have red faces, clenched jaws, and look totally spent when they finally put the weight down. All of this is fine, *if* you don't have fibromyalgia. This kind of weight lifting is a sure bet to trigger pain, and that's exactly what we're trying to eliminate with exercise, not cause.

If you are still unsure whether you are working hard enough without doing too much, think of the 1 to 10 scale. If 10 is the person with the red face and clenched jaw, and 2 is someone who barely looks like they are exercising, you want to be around an 8. You'll know you're an 8 in a couple of ways. First, your muscle will get weaker as you continue to lift the weight. Second, you'll feel a warm burning sensation in the muscle being worked. Third, you won't feel like you just burst a vital organ. You should feel like you are working hard, not like you're giving birth.

If following the beginner guidelines triggers a flare, stop lifting weights at once. Do not try to push through it. Focus on activity and stretching, along with the other things that help your flares.

Once the flare fades, you should figure out what triggered it. It may seem that the weight lifting triggered it, but if your sleep is not up to par, then that may have been the culprit. If your sleep is good, see if you can pinpoint exactly which exercise is causing problems. If you can point to one specific movement, double-check your form or substitute for it a different exercise. If you are not able to figure out exactly which exercises are aggravating things for you, eliminate all muscle conditioning for the parts of your body where you have the most pain. For example, if the majority of your pain is in your neck and shoulder area, avoid lifting weights that target this part of your body until you figure out what's going on. You may want to get some bodywork done on those hot spots; for more on this topic, see Chapter 7.

The Exceptions to the Rule

There will be individuals who never find a way to do muscle conditioning without causing recurrent flares. But I encourage you to not go down without a fight. The benefits of muscle conditioning are too important to simply give it up without really trying to find a way to make it work. But if you believe you've given it your best shot and it just isn't working out, I hope you can still feel good about your efforts to take wonderful care of yourself.

A word about soreness. It is normal to feel sore and a little stiff 24 to 48 hours after you start doing muscle conditioning. It is not normal to feel like you've been in a car accident. If you follow the guidelines outlined above, the soreness should be tolerable. In addition, as you get more fit, the postworkout soreness tends to go away and not come back unless you are really pushing yourself. There's a difference between the pain from normal muscle soreness and a fibromyalgia flare. With normal soreness, the muscle hurts mainly when you move it. It feels very similar to the last couple of times you lifted the weight as you exercised, and it feels immediately better when you rest the muscle.

I'm sure you're familiar with flare-type soreness. The key differences are that flare pain is constant, is often felt throughout your body, and doesn't go away when you stop flexing the muscle. Flare pain is hard to point to. Normal soreness is not. You can point to exactly the place it hurts, and it doesn't hurt anywhere else.

Now that you understand the difference between these kinds of pain, let me complicate things a bit. You can have both at the same time. As you start lifting weights it's possible that you may have normal conditioning-related pain along with your usual day-to-day pain. This is one of the reasons it's important to gradually increase your movement and to do so in the order presented in this book. If you were to start out with no activity, no stretching, and no aerobic conditioning, and launch yourself into weight lifting, you would need to make pain control a full-time job, if it wasn't already. By the time you get to muscle conditioning you should be ready for it, and this type of layered pain should be minimal. If you experience a little pain, you can simply treat it for what it is.

Conditioning-related soreness is usually helped by stretching and gentle activity. Heat and massage can also help, as can over-the-counter pain relievers. You'll want to wait for your next round of muscle conditioning until nearly all of the soreness has faded, which will be a few days.

Managing a fibromyalgia flare is covered more thoroughly later on, but whatever you do, don't lie down and hope it passes! By now I'm hoping you know that this causes more pain, not less. The good news is that much of what helps the soreness after lifting weights will also help flare pain. Remember to go slowly and gently, and to listen to your body.

The biggest mistakes made by people with fibromyalgia when they lift weights are either not trying muscle conditioning at all or refusing to modify the standard recommendations to their condition. Don't make these mistakes.

In Review

Do not attempt any muscle conditioning if your sleep quality is poor or if you are not already getting regular aerobic exercise and activity. If you are not already stretching, you should start before you attempt muscle conditioning.

Muscle conditioning can be done at home or in a gym. Regardless of where you choose to do it, be sure you have a trainer teach you how to lift weights or a reliable videotape to watch.

It's critical that you use proper form when lifting weights.

Do not use traditional exercise guidelines to lift weights if you have fibromyalgia. Use the guidelines in this book.

CHAPTER 7

Knowing When to Rest

You may be surprised that I advocate rest in this book because I spend so much time encouraging movement. Rest, however, is a crucial part of movement. If that sounds like convoluted logic to you, then you have something to learn from rest.

What do you think of when you hear the word *rest*? Do you picture yourself turning into a flabby TV junkie if you allow yourself to rest? Does rest seem overly self-indulgent to you? Maybe you let your body rest, but your mind is chattering at you the whole time with lists of things you should be doing. Do you rest only when you are in extreme pain, thinking to yourself, "I should keep going since I feel okay right now? There's no telling when I'll be incapacitated again." Is it possible that continually pushing yourself and refusing to rest might be *causing* the incapacitation? Could it be that making more moderate and balanced choices might reduce your pain? If these questions are starting to make you wonder more about rest, read on.

Many people have what's called all-or-nothing thinking. This means that you can toss any topic at them and you'll get an all-or-nothing way of looking at it. You can ask one woman why she doesn't exercise and she'll say, "I don't have any time." Ask another why she doesn't take a day off to rest and she'll roll her eyes and say, "If I stop moving, I'll never start again." This is all-or-nothing thinking.

Do you sometimes experience all-or-nothing thinking? Have you ever heard yourself say, "Well, I missed one day of exercise, so now I've messed it all up. There's no point in continuing"? Or maybe you're familiar with, "I can't exercise five days a week, so what's the point? Two days a week won't do anything for me." If this is starting to sound familiar, you're not alone.

All-or-nothing thinking keeps you from taking care of yourself because you are more focused on why you *can't* do something than on how you *can* do it. It makes you say, "Yes, but..." to every suggestion. If you find yourself saying, "Yes, but..." a lot, or if your friends and family are getting burned out from supporting you, there's a good chance you do some all-or-nothing thinking.

Knowing when to rest requires that you let go of all-or-nothing thinking. Balancing rest and movement instead of taking either one to extremes will help your pain most. Rest and movement work best together; each one enhances the other. When you move regularly, you rest better. And if you rest when you need to, you can move better.

From the perspective of fibromyalgia and exercise, you will need to pay close attention to your pain and its possible triggers. If you are spending a day inside reading or watching TV and your pain is increasing as the day goes on, you need to move. When you start to feel your muscles stiffen, you need to move. When you are restless and stiff or have been spending more than 30 minutes in one position, you need to move. It doesn't even matter what you do, just get up and move: check on the kids or pet, refill your water glass, make yourself some tea, or straighten up around the house.

This is the point at which most people with fibromyalgia will reach for pain relief in pill form. Most of the time you'll never need to reach for those pills if you get up and move. Give it at least 10 minutes of moving around and stretching before you take anything. When you have fibromyalgia, movement is like a pain relieving medicine.

If, on the other hand, you are hanging wallpaper and your pain is increasing as the day goes by, you need to rest. If you are lifting large bags of soil and wheelbarrows full of bark chips and are starting to feel like you've been hit by a truck, you need to rest. Intense movements like these push you out of the range of gentle movement and can trigger a flare. It does not mean you should stop moving completely. In fact, that's usually a big mistake. It means you should stop doing the movement that's causing you pain and ask for help in completing the task.

Getting the Rest You Need

For many of you, asking for help is difficult for a variety of reasons. I've had many clients tell me that asking for help means acknowledging that there's really something wrong with them, which is a reality they've been trying to avoid. Others have said they fear being rejected by family members and being told to stop acting helpless. These feelings are completely understandable. No one wants to have fibromyalgia, and certainly no one wants to be told they are acting helpless when they take a risk and ask for help. Nevertheless, the reality remains that there really *is* something wrong with you. Fibromyalgia is a real condition.

If you refuse to take care of yourself, it will be harder for people to support you. I had a client who refused to stop doing the things that were sure to trigger her pain flares. It was almost as if she was daring the fibromyalgia to affect her and desperately trying to prove there wasn't anything wrong with her. After two years of constant pain, she was depressed and at risk of being laid off from her job, largely because her performance and attendance were poor because of the chronic pain. She was furious and thought that she was being discriminated against because she had fibromyalgia. She failed to see that if she had taken care of herself and managed her condition, her boss wouldn't have had any problems with her performance. If you aren't willing to take care of yourself, you can't expect others to do it for you. And you can't blame them when your health deteriorates and starts limiting your ability to function.

Another client of mine was stubborn about taking care of her condition because she didn't want to appear weak. "Besides," she reasoned, "it's just pain. It's not like I'm making myself any worse." She was making a big mistake about the long-term effects of chronic pain. Chronic pain, in addition to making your life miserable, can have far-reaching implications on your health.

Being in chronic pain is a state of stress on the body, and chronic stress leads to all kinds of problems. Some of these stress-related problems are clinical depression, anxiety disorders (such as panic attacks), poor immune functioning (which means more than just more colds and sore throats; your immune system also tackles cancer and other serious illnesses), an increase in your risk for heart disease and stroke, an increase in your cholesterol levels and blood pressure, and so on. You don't *have* to ask for help. But why wouldn't you want to? Don't refuse to rest in the name of kidding yourself that you're cured.

Occasionally I come across a person with fibromyalgia who seems to use the pain and fatigue of fibromyalgia as a way to avoid things he or she is clearly capable of doing. One woman I worked with seemed more interested in *acting* as though she was doing everything she could to manage her condition than in following through on the most important ways to help herself. She refused to move more than absolutely necessary. She was significantly overweight, refused to try anything to help her sleep, and worked the third shift at her job. She spent nearly all 24 hours of the day sedentary, oftentimes in one position with poor posture for hours on end. She believed she needed to receive disability benefits, and if she seemed able to handle her daily life, her doctor would never sign the necessary papers. By meeting with me, she seemed to be making an effort to get better. She'd say to me, "Nothing helps me. I've been talking to you for three months and my pain is still the same. I guess I have no choice but to go on disability." All her missed appointments, unfinished homework, and empty promises of "I'll try" were about staying sick, not getting better. I'm not saying this woman may not have needed disability. Only her doctor can determine that. I *am* saying that if she had moved more, she would have felt better. She's a perfect example of how too much rest can be just as bad as not enough.

There's no doubt that chronic pain conditions like fibromyalgia affect your family members, and these people can react in a variety of ways. But if you are serious in caring for fibromyalgia, you will need to risk a family member's reaction and ask for help.

With any request, how you ask for what you need matters as much as what you ask for. People aren't mind readers, and you'll need to be specific. Saying, "None of you care about me! I'd have to be half dead to get any help around here" is different than saying, "I'm not sure if you realize it or not, but hanging this wallpaper border is going to kill my neck. If I wet down and prep the paper, will you hang it? I'd really appreciate it."

I know some of you are in an environment where there is a real chance of being emotionally or verbally abused if you ask for help, no matter how respectfully the request is voiced. Only you can decide if it seems safe enough to try, but I encourage you to give those that love you a chance. It's not fair to you or them if you are upset because they haven't read your mind or seem uncaring. Unless you are really making slaves out of your family, no one will think you are lazy, unreasonable, or helpless.

Sometimes you need to move, and other times you need to rest. If you know a certain task is too difficult and have tried to be clear about your needs and still get no response, you need to find another way to rest without the help of that person. Is there someone else in the household who could help you? Do you have a neighbor, friend, or other relative who could lend a hand on occasion? If taking care of yourself is a priority, you will find a way.

There will certainly be times when you may need to deal with a situation and handle the pain later. If your basement is flooding and it's just you and one other person there to haul heavy buckets of water to a drain, then you'll be hauling water. I'm not suggesting you say, "Oh, I'm sorry. I can't help you save our house and belongings. I need to rest so I don't trigger a flare." You'll have to manage the flare after the crisis is over.

What Rest Is and Is Not

It is important that I mention what rest is *not*. Rest is not time spent criticizing yourself for not doing more; "I really should be steam-cleaning the carpets," or "I shouldn't be taking this time to walk during my lunch break, there's still so much to do" doesn't qualify as rest. It's better than pushing yourself to steam-clean the carpets or skipping your midday walk, but it's not full rest. You need to do more than *act* as if you're resting. You need to *feel* as if you're resting. There's a very different physiologic state between the two. If you are seething with resentment over a disagreement with your boss and spend your walk picturing ways to get back at him or her, you are likely to return to your desk in more pain than when you left because you never actually rested. Rest is also not sleeping all day or spending long periods of time reading or watching TV.

Rest is taking a break at the start of a pain flare. It's saying, "I can't sit at this desk another minute. I need to get up and move for a while." Rest is allowing yourself to move gently and not pushing yourself through exercise. Rest is having the assertiveness to say, "I'm really sorry but I can't help you finish lifting all these boxes into your new apartment. Give me a few minutes to stretch and relax, and then I'd like to walk up to the corner store and get everyone a snack."

What if I'm Sick or Injured?

I'm often asked how much rest is appropriate during an illness or after surgery. The answer depends on how much pain you can stand.

For someone without fibromyalgia, having a bad cold might mean staying home from work, lying on the couch all day, and getting up only to manage the most urgent bodily functions.

Because you are a person with fibromyalgia, you will need to make a few changes to this routine if you want to avoid a full-blown flare. Unless you are completely knocked out from an illness, try to keep your time spent motionless to 30 minutes. Get up and refill your water glass, take a shower, stretch, and move around the house doing light activity. If someone is available, have him or her rub your neck and shoulders. Avoid being waited on for your every need unless you really need it. Being sick is bad enough. Being sick *and* dealing with fibromyalgia pain is even worse. Chronic pain will drain your body's energy to recover from whatever you are fighting. This isn't the time to pop an exercise tape into the VCR or go to the gym to lift weights, but it will help if you get some activity and do some stretching.

The advice is similar if you are recovering from surgery. Let your doctor know that you are concerned about managing your fibromyalgia during your hospital stay and after you return home. The process of surgery often triggers nasty flares. The position of your body during the surgery, the tendency of your body to respond to trauma with solidified soft tissue, and the emotional stress of surgery can send any person with fibromyalgia over the edge. To help make the whole experience more comfortable, plan ahead by telling your doctor(s) that you are concerned about a flare and see if you can have an order for medication ready in case you need it. Make arrangements to have a close friend or family member massage any areas that have become painful. If you wear a mouth guard at night to keep your face muscles relaxed bring it with you if you are staying overnight. A little planning will go a long way.

Once you leave the hospital, you'll want to know exactly what you can and can't do. Tell your doctor you want to do as much as is safely possible, as soon as possible. It helps if you can describe what you want to do so your doctor can approve it. Luckily, walking and moving around the house is safe almost immediately after many procedures. Even the day after major heart surgery, most patients are up and moving around. If your doctor approves this kind of movement, make full use of it. Be sure to ask if mild stretching is allowed, and if so, whether there are stretches you will need to avoid. Be sure to ask when you can return to exercise and to doing other movements you might be using to care for the fibromyalgia, and get back into your normal routine as soon as it's safe to do so.

If you need to do an extended stay in the hospital (more than one or two days) you definitely do not want to have a fibromyalgia pain flare in addition to everything else. Be clear with your nurses about needing to get up as often as possible and why. Even if you don't go any farther than to the bathroom and then sit in a nearby chair for a little while, do so. Stretch as much as you reasonably can, even while in bed. Ask the nurses to show you some simple stretches that can be done in bed. You'll have to ask for this kind of information. It's no secret that nurses and other hospital staff are incredibly busy, and as a result, this kind of care is not typically addressed in the hospital. You'll need to bring it up if you want less pain.

Plan Ahead for Less Pain

One of the clear messages of this book is to be proactive. After years of mysterious, stubborn pain, it's very easy to start feeling powerless with fibromyalgia. But once you know what works, you can make a plan when faced with a new or challenging situation. Most of the time, that plan will include time set aside for both rest and movement.

By balancing rest and movement, you can avoid too much of either, which can trigger pain. A body that gets balanced exercise, activity, sleep, recovery time, nutrition, work, and love feels relaxed, healthy, strong, and fulfilled. This can be you. Keep this image in your mind and heart. Make use of the resources you have while you learn to create new ones. It *is* possible.

Sophie was always in motion. She moved from the minute that her feet hit the floor in the morning until she collapsed at night. She had long since learned that her pain improved when she moved, and she hasn't stopped since.

For Sophie, rest meant doing only one task at a time. She was always doing at least two things at once. At work, she'd talk on the phone while reading her e-mails and eating lunch. At home, she'd make dinner while listening to the news and reading the mail.

The only time she stopped moving was when she was asleep or sick. And both were sure to generate pain. It was at the point that she couldn't even read a magazine without stiffening up like a brittle clay pot. She had begun to fear rest, thinking it caused the pain.

While searching the Internet, Sophie learned that her inability to relax could be causing the pain. She noticed that when she sat down to watch TV she felt so restless she had to get up and do something while she watched. The Internet article said if you couldn't remember the last time you felt deeply, completely relaxed, you knew you had at least one of your pain triggers identified.

Sophie tried to remember the last time she was totally relaxed. Her mind spiraled backwards, searching for a recollection of complete bliss. Even while on vacation she made lists of things to see and do and was always in perpetual motion. It seemed a resting place was always around some future corner.

Sophie was realizing that learning to rest would be no easy task. It would mean leaving things undone, trying to quiet the chatter in her mind, and learning to sit still.

She quickly realized that it was easier to relax when someone else controlled the environment and when her body was involved. She found that taking a walk and then a long, scented bath allowed her to lie still in her bed for a while. She made her bath extra restful by lighting the room with candles, playing soft music, and wearing her favorite robe afterward.

She also found that a professional massage was a guaranteed hour of relaxation. She came out of the therapist's office feeling warm from the inside out, totally relaxed and uncaring about any problem, no matter how urgent.

As she practiced relaxing, she found that it was increasingly easier to make it happen. She even found that when she was getting tense at work, just remembering the massage room would release her muscles. She got some of the lotion her massage therapist used, and she found the smell could trigger her body to relax. Sophie no longer fears her body.

In Review

To best care for fibromyalgia, you will need to balance your needs for rest and movement, which requires that you let go of all-or-nothing thinking.

Rest is not lying still while you obsess about stressful events.

Learn how to ask for help constructively.

If you aren't willing to take responsibility for your body, you can't blame doctors, medications, or other people for not curing you.

Plan ahead for new or challenging situations. Be proactive.

CHAPTER 8

Alternative Care for Fibromyalgia

Almost every fibromyalgia patient I've worked with has tried some alternative form of care. Many have tried treatments such as acupuncture or herbs, or other approaches to pain relief. Although the research examining how these interventions affect fibromyalgia is still in early stages, the anecdotal support for some of these forms of pain relief is growing. These reports and the early research look wonderfully promising in providing new ways to help manage fibromyalgia, but beware: some approaches can have little or no effect and will cost you valuable time and money.

What's a Person to Do?

I've heard many people, myself among them, complain that it's too hard to sort out what is fact and what is fiction in the world of complementary care. Due in part to the early stage of research on the topic and lack of regulation in nearly all areas of complementary care, most insurance companies are unwilling to pay for this kind of care, which leaves desperately hurting patients to toy with expensive, untested care.

The lack of research also makes many physicians feel less than fully informed about other ways to manage chronic pain, and they are therefore often reluctant to offer much enthusiasm if a patient has questions about complementary care. Physicians want to provide you with the most effective, safe, and reliable relief for your pain that's possible, but there's no way for them to know what is safe or effective.

In fact, there are still doctors who will tell patients that there is no such thing as fibromyalgia, that there is nothing that can be done, and to just learn to live with the pain. Patients, on the other hand, feel desperate to get some relief. After years of debilitating flares, limited lives, and failed treatments, is it any wonder we are willing to spend money and try anything to get some relief? The process of science can be slow, and there seems to be nowhere to get reliable information on what options are credible and which ones are a waste of money.

For the record, I am an ardent supporter of the scientific method. I'm very cautious of miracle cures with no evidence to support the claims, and you should be too. There are billions of dollars being spent and made in the alternative health care movement, and not all of those dollars are helping people get better. And to be sure, some of those dollars are hurting people. Of course, the same can be said of Western medicine, so there's something good to be said for being skeptical when it comes to your health.

Being skeptical is not the same as being cynical. Skeptics are open-minded and willing to change their behavior if the evidence supports doing so. Skeptics proceed with caution in all cases and want to be an informed part of any decision. They accept reasonable risk and take responsibility for their decisions and possible outcomes. Skeptics understand the reasoning in most cases for beginning with the least-invasive and least-expensive treatment and slowly moving toward more aggressive care.

Cynics assume ill intent and mistrust even when there is overwhelming evidence to the contrary. They are resistant to new information and will continue the same behavior regardless of whether it's beneficial.

Both patients and doctors can be cynics or skeptics. You should aim to be a skeptic and to suppress any tendency toward cynicism. And you want a medical provider, regardless of his or her professional training, to be the same.

There's an old saying, "Absence of evidence is not evidence of absence." Just because there is no evidence that a treatment will work doesn't mean that it won't. If a treatment has not been fully tested, it might work and it might not. You will have to proceed with caution and at your own risk.

Western medicine will need to integrate new ideas and ways of thinking, and the alternative world is in the process of combing through their claims to find which ones are supportable and which ones are not. If you have a doctor who tells you that nothing can be done for fibromyalgia, you aren't getting the best possible care. If you are paying $200 per month in nutritional supplements and can't feel a significant improvement, you are wasting your money. If after dozens of medical appointments, gallons of potions, and bottles of pills, someone asks you if you feel better, you should be able to give a clear answer. Responses like, "I think so," "A little," and "I can't tell" mean that it's time to try something else. But if you can say, "I'm definitely improved," or "Wow, what a difference!" or "I actually feel better" then you are on the right track.

How to Use Alternative Treatment

If you want to avoid wasting time and money, there is a very specific way to go about trying alternative forms of care. Be your own scientist. Following are some recommendations for considering any care, traditional or alternative, while we all wait for the day when there is no division between the two.

1. Start with your primary doctor first. Once you are connected to a doctor you trust, who is open to work with your desire for alternative care, listen to what options she or he recommends. If you expect them to be open with you, you need to be open to what they say.

2. Let your doctor know what you plan to try. Research on patients who use alternative care shows that the overwhelming majority don't tell their physicians about it. Don't let this be you. If you expect Western medicine to open up, you need to give honest feedback to its

practitioners about what has worked and what hasn't. A good doctor will be attentive to this.

3. Try only one new treatment at a time. Let's say you start medications in an effort to sleep better, and take herbs and a homeopathic remedy all in the same week. If you get better, how will you know what helped you? Are you planning to pay for, and continue to take, all these remedies forever? How will you know what treatment to stop first? When should you stop it? What if two or more treatments are working together to reduce the pain? The only way to know is to go slow.

4. Try the things we know work first. There is an abundance of research showing that several things help fibromyalgia pain. You should first try medications to help you sleep, get regular activity and exercise specifically designed for fibromyalgia, minimize long periods with no movement, and make sure the rest of you is healthy by maintaining a normal weight, eating properly, and not smoking. One patient of mine complained constantly about how nothing would help her pain and that all the doctors were mystified by her case. She had tried a long list of medications, supplements, and chiropractic and physical therapy care to no effect. She was just over 5 feet tall, weighed well over 200 pounds, smoked, didn't exercise, and was usually on some kind of diet that left her malnourished and famished. If you refuse to take care of yourself, don't blame the care providers or their treatments if you still feel lousy.

5. When starting a new treatment, use it *exactly* as you are told by the practitioner who recommended it or by the label on the bottle. If the treatment doesn't work, you won't know if it was ineffective for you or if you just didn't use it right. Ask questions, read about the treatment you are considering, and be sure you know how to do your part.

6. Give it time. Very few treatments offer immediate help. Although activity and stretching will help ease pain right

away, the full benefits of movement come after several weeks. Most herbs require that you take them for a few weeks before a noticeable effect is possible. Be realistic about your expectations while being responsible with your care.

7. Know who's treating you. Never allow someone to treat you without knowing anything about him or her. In addition to knowing what a practitioner's credentials are, you will want to check out his or her familiarity with fibromyalgia. If you are thinking about taking herbs, be sure to find a company that's reputable, as none of the herbal supplements are regulated at this time. This means you don't really know exactly what or how much is inside the bottle. Even if the amounts are listed on the label, there's no guarantee that it's accurate. Although reputable practitioners and companies exist, there are also many that are just out to take your money, and you'll have little recourse if you are harmed.

8. Be explicitly honest with yourself. If a treatment isn't working, admit it. If you've followed all the steps listed here, and a particular approach isn't helping, discontinue it. No matter how disappointed you are, how much money you've spent on it, how much you wanted it to work, and how hopeless you feel about what to do next, there's no point in continuing with something that isn't working. I know one woman with fibromyalgia who was spending $200 a month on supplements for over two years. Her pain was unchanged, and yet she continued to take them, hoping they'd start to help. If it hasn't helped in two years, it's not going to. Know when to stop.

Before I discuss the variety of other pain-relief options available, let me stress the importance of movement for pain relief. There *is* research showing that exercise can significantly help fibromyalgia. This is solid, controlled evidence that you can trust and invest in. Both Western and alternative healers agree completely on this point. By using movement, you are relying on your body's own healing system. You *know* you will respond to it. Everyone does, assuming it's done correctly. What's more, it's usually inexpensive, doesn't require you to swallow anything risky, and will improve your health in dozens of other ways in addition to easing your pain. If all that isn't enough, there's a good chance that the movement described in this book will enhance the effectiveness of other types of care.

Of all the available types of alternative care, there are a handful that have growing anecdotal claims of pain relief for fibromyalgia. Many of these treatments fall into the categories of both Western and alternative medicine. Some consider chiropractic care clearly in the realm of Western medicine, and others feel it is in the realm of alternative medicine. Some practitioners even refer to exercise and healthy eating as alternative! I wish I could say that the division between the two was easy to make. Unfortunately this is not the case. And much research will need to be done to determine the degree of benefit for various alternative treatments. I've chosen to exclude chiropractic care and physical therapy from this discussion because most physicians are familiar with them and there are established standards for certification, licensing, and best practice. In other words, the words *chiropractor* and *physical therapist* imply a specific level of skill and training.

This is different from titles such as massage therapist, acupuncturist, herbalist, and so on. Although this is changing, the progress is slow and limited to regional pockets across the United States. One state might license acupuncturists, and another might not. One person who recommends herbs might be called an herbalist, and another might be called a botanical healer.

For this chapter, I'm going to focus on several areas that are still clearly in the realm of alternative medicine and show early promise of easing the pain of fibromyalgia.

Bodywork

Bodywork can refer to a dizzying array of services. Practices developed over the centuries in different parts of the world all have different approaches to working things out via your body. Some of these are well-known, like sports massage, and others are less well-known but have devoted followings. Many of these styles of bodywork have developed very specific ways of dealing with the pain of fibromyalgia.

Several of these schools of thought incorporate techniques that involve locating painful tender points and trigger points and holding a constant pressure on them for several seconds. The technique has acquired a few different names, the most common being trigger-point release, pressure-point therapy, and fascicle release. This is not your usual relaxation massage, although some traditional massage techniques may be used between work on specific areas. The tender points and trigger points are, by definition, painful. So it's no surprise that pushing on them hurts. But doing so can provide incredible relief *if* you are also using movement as described in this book.

It's thought that this type of bodywork breaks up the tight fascicle lining covering the muscles that can restrict movement and make you feel stiff. It also seems to relieve spasms and scar tissue that may be in, or on, the muscle tissue. It may also be that this type of pain stimulus may cause your nervous system to not feel the other pain.

Regardless of how it works, it seems to reduce pain for many people, *if* they do their part to move when and how they need to. If after visiting your massage therapist you go home and read for the rest of the day, you are still going to have plenty of pain from inactivity. But if you continue to move in the ways discussed in this book, then there's a good chance you'll have less pain overall and for extended periods of time.

Exercise can help enhance the effects of alternative care. If you are in less pain, you will feel more like moving. If you move more, you will have less pain. Bodywork can greatly improve your ability to do the other things that will help keep you free of pain.

If you find that this technique works well for you, ask your therapist how to do it on yourself! There are many parts of your body that you can reach, and a good therapist will be happy to teach you how to do it correctly.

Biofeedback

Chronic pain usually leads to chronic muscle tension. And chronic muscle tension leads to more pain. The cycle becomes unending, and the pain can be completely debilitating.

This is especially true with fibromyalgia because pain sensations tend to be intensified by the condition. After weeks and months of constant pain, muscles you never knew you had might be screaming for release. It's thought that this is part of why so many people with fibromyalgia also have facial pain and temporomandibular disorders. This kind of pain can be baffling to your medical providers. They can't find anything wrong with you, yet you are incapacitated by pain.

As the research about chronic pain grows, a new type of healer has emerged: a healer trained in using conscious will to control pain and who also has first-rate skills to help patients cope with chronic illness. This type of provider is often a licensed psychologist with special training in mind-body interaction and knows a variety of ways of making fibromyalgia easier to cope with.

Among their methods is a technique called biofeedback. With biofeedback, you use cues from your body to help you change your behavior. When you get full, you stop eating. When you are cold, you put on a sweater. When you feel stiff, you get up and move. These are all forms of biofeedback.

There are subtle changes you can make that can dramatically change the pain. The process is simply putting a sensor on your skin that reads muscle tension on a dial that resembles a gas gauge, which is placed in front of you. When your muscle tension is high, it will tell you by moving the indicator needle to the right. When you relax your muscles, the needle falls back to the left.

When you are in chronic pain, many muscles start to hold tension that you are not aware of. The dial allows you to get immediate feedback about when they are relaxed, so you can memorize the feeling and re-create it outside the office.

No one is saying that the pain is all in your head. Biofeedback just helps you use your attention to affect your body. You will need to practice the technique between visits, and as always, your progress is more up to you than your provider. It's hard to over-estimate the impact biofeedback can have on chronic pain.

Not surprisingly, exercise and other forms of movement greatly enhance your ability to learn and master biofeedback tech-niques. Fit people are more in touch with their bodies and have more resources to draw from to affect it. They have better volun-tary muscle control, are more relaxed, and have an easier time relaxing than their nonfit counterparts. Exercise will enhance biofeedback, and biofeedback will help you feel better so you can move more.

If you are interested in trying biofeedback, you can ask your doctor if she or he can refer you to a good practitioner.

Herbs

I'm often asked which herbal supplements help fibromyalgia. I'm not an expert on herbal medicine, but I've seen enough patients get better using herbal supplements as a part of their care plan to convince me there's a place for it.

Herbs seem to help symptoms of fibromyalgia when used to improve quality of sleep and reduce muscle tension. If you are interested in experimenting, start asking around to find a good supplier of herbs and recommendations of which ones to try. Remember to take the herb exactly as directed for at least a month. Be sure you know the potential side effects and interac-tions with other medications, and let your doctor know what you're doing. Use just one herb at a time or you won't know which ones are causing a change.

At the risk of sounding like a broken record, herbs and exer-cise can complement each other and are best used together. If herbs are helping you sleep and decreasing your levels of muscle tension, then you will have more energy and less pain during and after exercise, which will allow you to do more and tolerate it better.

Cautious Optimism

Being cautiously open is a good approach when it comes to your health and healing, regardless of what methods you are using. Ask for explanations of what you're being told. There are many ways to connect with and heal your body. There are also many ways to lose your faith in healing, along with a lot of cash, by turning your body over to someone not qualified to take care of it.

Jennifer felt hopeless. She had been to countless doctors and healers and taken bottles full of pills. Nothing seemed to ease the pain. Her fibromyalgia had been diagnosed four years earlier, and at age 49, she felt like it was only going to get worse. Years of chronic pain and seeing stumped doctors left her wondering if she could live another year like this. She avoided spending any energy outside of her efforts to survive her day-to-day pain. She was so exhausted from enduring constant pain that she went to bed early every night to lie on a heating pad and wait for her prescription muscle relaxants to take effect. She had forgotten what normal and happy feel like.

A coworker of Jennifer's who also had fibromyalgia gave her the name of her doctor and encouraged her to make an appointment. Jennifer wasn't sure she had the energy to tell the whole story again to someone new, but she couldn't think of anything that she had to lose.

Jennifer told her story to the new physician, who listened closely. Afterward, the doctor explained that chronic pain has an eroding effect on many different parts of the body and that depression is one way this erosion can show up. She explained how stress affects the neurotransmitters in the brain, making depression almost a certainty. She encouraged Jennifer to try a second medication in addition to the one she was already taking to help her sleep, and then gave her specific advice on how to use exercise to ease the pain. Jennifer asked the doctor about massage, and although the doctor wasn't familiar with its use with fibromyalgia, she agreed it couldn't hurt her.

Jennifer felt reluctant to have hope again, but she didn't see any alternative. She agreed to try the second medication, and within two weeks she started to notice a change. Her energy level was higher than it had been in months. The pain had improved, and she no longer felt like she was living in a dark hole.

She pulled out the information on exercise the doctor had given her. She had never thought of herself as an exerciser, but what the doctor described was very mild. She started by doing the stretches pictured on the handouts. Her muscles and joints felt better immediately. After a week of stretching three times a day, she started taking short walks in the morning and evening. During the second walk, she noticed that while she was walking she had no pain at all! She couldn't remember the last time she felt so wonderful!

She met with her new doctor four weeks later to check in on her progress. She described what she had done and how much it helped. Her doctor commended her on the fine job of self-care she had done and suggested she see the health psychologist at the clinic for biofeedback training.

Jennifer had never realized that she could control so much about her body. The psychologist taught her how to relax, something Jennifer had long forgotten how to do. Soon Jennifer was able to keep her muscle tension readings in the normal range and was beginning to feel her life might include more than just pain. It was quite a revelation to Jennifer that emotional tension could translate so directly into body pain. Now she understands that pain can be used to signal that she needs to center herself and relax. Jennifer feels like she's back in control of her body.

In Review

Whether considered alternative or conventional, regular activity and exercise combined with healthy eating and quality sleep are the most important treatments for fibromyalgia.

For help with pain and other symptoms, there are other forms of healing that show great promise.

Some types of care, both alternative and conventional, are at best ineffective, most likely expensive, and at worst dangerous. Proceed with caution.

For any new treatment, follow the guidelines in this book for the best chance of relief and self-protection.

Be willing to admit when a treatment has not worked for you.

CHAPTER 9

Managing Flares

There's no question about it. A fibromyalgia flare is painful and sometimes completely debilitating. It can eclipse every aspect of your life and demand all of your attention.

Most people have tried many things to manage flares. Although what works for one person might not work for another, there are definitely some common things that will help anyone experiencing a flare.

There are two main goals in managing a flare. First, you need to deal with the acute pain. Second, you need to figure out what triggered it so you can avoid it in the future. I've found it helpful to distinguish between a minor and a major flare because they often require different strategies.

Minor flares last one to three days and do not require you to alter your normal routine in any way. This could be a nagging tension headache, tight hip muscles that make you walk a little funny, an increase in morning stiffness, and so on. You are still able to do whatever activities you had planned (including exercise), although you might be more tired than usual at the end of the day.

Major flares are longer lasting, life-altering monsters. If intense pain lasts longer than a few days, or comes on suddenly and keeps you from doing anything for the rest of the day, you're having a major flare. Under these circumstances, people go running for a quiet, dark room to rest in and hope to be put out of their misery.

The suggestions on page 106 should be helpful for managing both kinds of flares. Obviously, nothing is written in stone. This approach is based on my own clinical experience, not on extensive research. Use this as a guideline along with your good judgment and physician's input.

Managing Flares

For minor flares, try to do the following:

- Catch them early.
- Take a break from whatever you're doing.
- Get some gentle movement (such as a short walk).
- Stretch, focusing on the most painful areas while breathing deeply.
- Relax. Although it's normal to tense up when you are in pain, it only makes it worse.
- Drink some water and have a small snack.
- Have someone massage the tight area (or possibly do it yourself).
- Make sure you get an especially good night's sleep.

Try to avoid the following:

- Taking any medications unless specifically directed by your doctor.
- Remaining in the same position or doing the same activity that triggered the pain.
- Tension-creating thoughts ("I just know this is going to escalate into a horrendous flare!").
- Getting too hungry or thirsty.
- Caffeine.
- Anything else that might increase your muscle tension (such as bright sunlight, loud music, uncomfortable clothing or furniture).

Minor flares respond well to activity and stretching. Taking medication to manage this type of flare can cause problems due to a phenomenon called rebound pain. Rebound pain occurs when your body responds to frequent doses of pain relievers (such as ibuprofen) by increasing the pain as soon as the medication wears off. Many fibromyalgia patients are stunned to learn that frequent or excessive use of pain relievers may actually be *causing* the pain they feel after the last dose wore off. This is why it's so important to not use them for minor flares. You'll do better if you use movement to handle it.

Major flares, on the other hand, are so incapacitating that it's hard to imagine doing much of anything. It's often necessary to get some help at the onset of a major flare, and once the pain has eased up a little, use the suggestions I provided for the minor flares. During a major flare, try to do the following:

- Clear your schedule for the rest of the day.
- Take whatever medications reliably help you in this situation with 8 to 16 ounces of water.
- Get some hands-on healing. If you have a massage therapist, see if it's possible to be seen on short notice.
- Find the most comfortable position you can with as little stimulus as possible (low light, quiet room).
- Use a heating pad or take a hot bath.
- Stay calm and reassure yourself. "The medication will kick in in a few minutes. I have the whole evening to just take care of myself. I know the heat will feel wonderful."

Try to avoid the following:

- Ignoring the pain. Your body is screaming for relief. Don't try and force yourself to keep going.
- Anything physical. When you are in this kind of shape, any movement is interpreted by your body as stress and causes you to tighten up even more. Don't go to the gym in this condition, unless, of course, you're going for a massage or to sit in the whirlpool.
- Eating. You will likely be lying down, and you won't want a full belly. Also, when the body is in this much pain it's not

uncommon to feel nauseated, and the last thing you want to do is vomit.

- All stimuli. No phones, people, or pets. No TV, radio, or talking. The obvious exception to this would be a massage therapist or other person helping to relieve the pain.
- Feeling guilty or like a burden to those helping you.

Once the pain subsides, you can start thinking about what triggered such a major flare. When I'm working with a patient who can't get the flares under control, here's what I recommend he or she do, in this order.

1. Stop doing all muscle conditioning and aerobic exercise except for water aerobics and walking.
2. Maintain lots of stretching and daily activity.
3. Evaluate your sleep. If you have any reason to think you are not sleeping as well as you should be, see your doctor as soon as possible and make any needed changes.
4. If there are no remaining sleep problems, begin looking at each part of your day. What might you be doing to aggravate certain hot spots on your body? Is there a certain time of day that you have the most pain? What are you doing right before the pain is at its worst?
5. Evaluate your basic health practices. Are you eating as well as you could be? Might you need nutritional supplements? Do you smoke? What is your posture like at work? In the car? At home? Is part of your exercise routine to blame?
6. Take some time every day to deeply relax. If you have difficulty doing this, get some help such as biofeedback training.

It's easy to start getting used to chronic pain and to forget what it feels like to be without it. It's crucial to not let that happen and to take flares seriously. Chronic pain is not normal. Living a blunted life is not acceptable. It *is* possible for you to take control of fibromyalgia and live a normal life.

In Review

Minor and major flares may require slightly different approaches.

Unless you are truly incapacitated by the flare, try to use movement to reduce the pain.

If used too often, medications can actually worsen fibromyalgia pain by causing rebound pain.

If flares are frequent or severe, return to the basics of sleep, movement, and bodywork for relief and prevention of future problems.

CHAPTER 10

Putting It All Together

This book contains a lot of information. While you were reading, I hope you found many places where you could make changes and have less pain. If you are drowning in information and are still unsure of how to put it all together in a way that will reduce the pain and still leave you with time to live your life, I'm sure you're not alone. Each of us must experiment to find the right balance that meshes with our lives, bodies, and resources. No one expects the final picture to be the same for everyone. Only you can decide what works.

This chapter will offer you different pictures of health. Each person is managing his or her fibromyalgia well, but most have changes still to be made. No one is cured. Most were willing to move more, and differently, than they had been. Hopefully you are too.

Remember to start with activity and build from there. If you have fibromyalgia and don't have time to get regular activity, you have no business lifting weights. Unless you feel very confident that you can manage any messy results, don't try to do other forms of exercise without activity.

There is almost certainly a lot going on in your life. There is no way that any one person can do everything suggested here, so don't try. The best way to use this book, or any other self-help book for that matter, is to notice what single change you feel drawn to make first (or next) and begin working out the details of how to make it happen. The following questions and tips have been adapted from the Transtheoretical Model of Behavior Change, which was created by James Prochaska. (Incidentally, Stages of Change, developed by Prochaska, works for any change you might be considering. Whether you change your brand of laundry detergent, begin exercising, or buy a house, the same stages are necessary.) If this approach interests you, Prochaska's work is listed at the end of the book. For the rest of you, the following questions and suggestions will get at the same information.

Thinking about Change

1. Write down *one* change you are thinking about making. You do not need to have already committed to it, but it does need to be specific. For example, if you wrote "exercise," it's going to be nearly impossible to work out the details because the change is too broad. And although "ride my bike four times a week, stretch twice a day, and lift weights three days a week" is specific, it's *way* too much change. Those of you who think of yourselves as go-getters won't like this, but I recommend not making more than one significant change every three to six months. And every time you add a new change, you are at increased risk for sliding on the most recent one, so go slow and use the questions here to help you.
   "I am thinking about ... _____
   _____."

2. Next, make a thorough list of the pros and cons of making the change. I've always liked the method of taking a clean sheet of paper, drawing a line down the center, and labeling one side "Pros" and the other "Cons." Here's the catch: according to Prochaska, the list of pros needs to be at least *twice* as long as the cons. So if your pro list is coming up short, don't move on until you've found some other reasons. It makes a real difference when we get a little further in the process.

3. Next, assuming you still want to make the change, you'll need to work out the logistical issues. Don't

skip this step or you'll fall off the wagon right away.
This crucial step is often missed and is a key reason
people don't keep up with a new behavior, no matter
how beneficial it is. This step is thinking the change
through and noticing all the little things you need to
have in place. If the change you want to make is to
get more aerobic exercise and you are planning to
start by walking during your lunch break at work,
there are certain things to consider. Do you need to
bring a special pair of walking shoes to work? Will
you want a change of clothes? If you want to wash
your face afterward, do you have the cleanser at work
that you need? Which days will you walk? Are you
walking alone or with someone else, and if so, with
whom? Do you need to schedule the time in your
appointment book, or is your day flexible enough
that you can go at your leisure? Similarly, if you are
thinking about getting more activity in your day,
there are also things to consider. Do you know where
the stairs are in the buildings that you normally
spend time in? Are the stairwells safe? If you park farther away from your destinations, how far are you
willing to walk? Do you have an umbrella in your
car? How will you make sure you have the extra time
it will take to walk from the farthest parking space? If
these issues are not solved, they'll be the first reason
you get off track. You can't plan for everything, but
plan for everything that you can.

4. Once you feel reasonably confident that you have
   considered the possible obstacles to your change, you
   need to pick a start date. Be realistic about the start
   date. Just because you presently have the plan in place
   doesn't always mean it is a good time to start. You
   may want to wait until after a doctor appointment,
   until a certain project at work is done, or after your
   favorite baby-sitter is out of school. Be sure to give

yourself time to resolve whatever potential problems you identified in step 3 when you choose the date.

5. Once the day has come, you are very vulnerable to simply reverting back to your old way of doing things. To help prevent this, it's important that you be willing to give your new change some special attention for a couple of weeks. This may mean checking in with a friend or family member to talk about how it's going. It may also mean setting aside some extra time until you develop a routine. Whatever it takes, plan for it and remember it won't take this level of mental energy forever. Keep your eyes open for new roadblocks that threaten your progress and deal with them right away. If maintaining the new behavior is turning out to feel like a full-time job, or if you can't keep it up, you'll need to go back to step one and start again. Usually change fails because the change was too broad, too complex, or the pro/con ratio wasn't at least 2:1.

6. Once you have kept up the new behavior for over six months with no significant slips, you can begin to shift your focus. Instead of paying attention to all the day-to-day obstacles, you can just think about the big ones that might come up once or twice a year, such as the holidays, a vacation, a minor injury or illness, boredom, and so on. If you feel very confident that you can deal with these obstacles with little or no risk of getting off track, you're ready to think about a new change, if you wish.

This process can be incredibly useful at guiding you through a change, and it's just as helpful at keeping you from wasting time if you really aren't ready. If I'm not sure a patient is really ready for a healthy change, I have him or her make a pro/con list. (Incidentally, a dead giveaway that someone isn't ready is if I hear things like, "I really *should* exercise," "I know I shouldn't be working an overnight shift, but…," or "If only I didn't have fibromyalgia, I'd get more activity.") Invariably, the list of cons is longer than the pros, and if that 2:1 ratio isn't there, I encourage the patient to hold off until he or she has really thought it through. What are you thinking about changing next? What does your list look like? Following are some examples of how real people have used this process successfully to manage fibromyalgia.

Megan was thinking about lifting weights. She already walked seven days a week, stretched twice a day, and got lots of daily activity at work. She tried several times to start a weight-lifting routine but kept getting stuck and overwhelmed. I had her complete a pro/con list and here's what we found:

Pro: I would look more toned.
Con: I can't afford the gym membership or videotapes and I hate lifting weights. The only way to make time would be to walk less, see my family less, or get up at 4 A.M. I'm always sore afterwards.

After looking at the lists, it was clear to both Megan and me why she was having trouble. Since her pain was in good control, and she was not overweight and otherwise healthy, I asked her what she thought about not trying to fit it in right now. She gave me the look I've come to recognize as meaning, "That never occurred to me, but I sure like the sound of it."

In case you are like Megan and need permission to comfortably choose to *not* do something that might be good for you, you have my permission. Sometimes that's the healthiest choice to make. The next example shows how the process worked for a different situation.

Jamie needed help getting started with aerobic exercise. After some work, she got her pro/con list to about a 4:1 ratio and really felt ready. She wanted to start that day, in fact, as soon as we were done with the session. At the end, I dropped the bombshell. "What do you need to have in place before you can start this?"

She paused a moment and then said she couldn't think of anything. I prodded a little further. "When you leave here, what are you going to do for exercise?" She had planned to go for a bike ride. "That's great," I said. "What about the day after that?" Jamie admitted that she hadn't thought that far ahead but that she would like do a combination of walking, biking, and swimming at her local pool. I asked her if everything she needed to make this happen was already in place. I could see she realized what she had to do, after some pondering. She began making a list of several things that, if dealt with now, would likely prevent her from failing in the next two weeks. She decided that by getting an extra pair of walking shoes to keep in her car, calling the county park for bike trail information, and prepacking a gym bag for use at the pool, she could make her exercise plan much more simple. She hit a couple of roadblocks along the way when the pool was closed for repair or the weather didn't cooperate, but after several months, she felt she was officially a regular exerciser.

A message that warrants repeating is to go slow. Give yourself the best possible chance to be successful at managing fibromyalgia and the rest of your life. You are human and have limitations. Make your choices carefully.

I encourage you to honor your individuality by honestly determining what your goal is and then to go about reaching it in whatever way you are most comfortable with. Be willing to ask for help and be open to trying something on your own. Be assertive with your medical care and scrupulously honest with yourself about what works and what doesn't. Get into the habit of listening to your body and trusting what it tells you. You do *not* have to accept chronic, debilitating pain from fibromyalgia. It is reasonable to expect that the pain can evolve from being a demonic force that controls your life to a signal that your body and mind need a change of some kind. It is reasonable to have the pain be tolerable and under your control.

It is essential, if you want less pain, that you move your body gently and carefully. Find the joy in movement and the connection to your body that may be the buried treasure you discover on this journey.

In Review

It's not possible to implement every suggestion in this book.

It's possible to manage fibromyalgia well without feeling as though your whole life is about the condition.

It is a realistic goal to have the pain of fibromyalgia under control.

There is a life outside of pain management.

Recommended Reading

Bailey, Covert. *The New Fit or Fat*. Boston: Houghton Mifflin Co., 1991.

———. *The Fit or Fat Woman*. Boston: Houghton Mifflin Co., 1989.

———. *Smart Exercise*. Boston: Houghton Mifflin Co., 1996.

Fransen, Jenny, and I. Jon Russell. *The Fibromyalgia Help Book: Practical Guide to Living Better with Fibromyalgia*. Minneapolis, Minn.: Chronimed Publishing, 1997.

Kabat-Zinn, Jon. *Full Catastrophe Living*. New York: Delta Books, 1990.

Louden, Jennifer. *The Woman's Comfort Book*. San Francisco: HarperSanFrancisco, 1992.

Prochaska, James. *Changing for Good*. New York: Avon Books, 1995.

Sapolsky, Robert M. *Why Zebras Don't Get Ulcers*. New York: W H Freeman and Co., 1998.

Starlanyl, Devin J. *Fibromyalgia and Chronic Myofascial Pain Syndrome: A Survival Manual*. Oakland, Calif.: New Harbinger Publications, 1996.

Index

About the Author

Stacie L. Bigelow, M.A., is a counselor, researcher, teacher, and writer. In addition to holding a master's degree in psychology, she has worked as a psychotherapist, health and fitness counselor, instructor and trainer, and care manager for many years. She is currently a counselor and research coordinator at HealthPartners in Minneapolis, Minnesota. She is an adjunct faculty member at the Adler Graduate School of Psychology. Stacie is the author and coauthor of over a dozen health-improvement courses and programs.